KU-698-027

Kitchen Solutions for Common Maladies

Sore Throats and Eye Trouble

Mix one ounce of quince seeds in a glass of boiling water and let stand for one hour. Strain. This solution is a useful eye drop for removing foreign matter and when mixed with an equal part of honey an hourly teaspoonful will relieve coughs and hoarseness.

Sprains and Bruises

Take coarse dry salt and heat in a pan. Put heated salt into heavy cloth material, such as a towel, and apply to sprained or bruised area.

Rashes

Mix ½ ounce brown soap, 2 ounces onion (roasted or steamed), 2 ounces dry ground mustard, 2 ounces sugar, and enough water to form a paste. Apply hot mixture to infected area within one or two days after rash has appeared. This ointment offers quick relief for itching and dermatitis due to poison ivy, poison oak, and poison sumac.

KITCHEN MEDICINES
was originally published by Barre Publishers.

*Are there paperbound books you want
but cannot find in your retail stores?*

You can get any title in print in **POCKET BOOK** editions. Simply send retail price, local sales tax, if any, plus 25¢ to cover mailing and handling costs to:

MAIL SERVICE DEPARTMENT
POCKET BOOKS • A Division of Simon & Schuster, Inc.
1 West 39th Street • New York, New York 10018

Please send check or money order. We cannot be responsible for cash. *Catalogue sent free on request.*

Titles in this series are also available at discounts in quantity lots for industrial or sales-promotional use. For details write our Special Projects Agency: The Benjamin Company, Inc., 485 Madison Avenue, New York, N.Y. 10022.

KITCHEN MEDICINES

by BEN CHARLES HARRIS

PUBLISHED BY POCKET BOOKS NEW YORK

KITCHEN MEDICINES

Barre edition published October, 1968

POCKET BOOK edition published June, 1970

5th printing........January, 1973

This POCKET BOOK edition includes every word
contained in the original, higher-priced edition. It is printed
from brand-new plates made from completely reset, clear, easy-to-read
type. POCKET BOOK editions are published by POCKET BOOKS, a division
of Simon & Schuster, Inc., 630 Fifth Avenue, New York, N.Y. 10020.
Trademarks registered in the United States and other countries.

L

Standard Book Number: 671-77534-0.
Library of Congress Catalog Card Number: 68-29794.
Copyright, ©, 1961, 1968, by Ben Charles Harris.
All rights reserved. This POCKET BOOK edition is published
by arrangement with Barre Publishers.

Printed in U.S.A.

To

The Members of the Health Club

Hobby and Museum Herb Clubs

ACKNOWLEDGMENT

I wish to express my gratitude to the scores of friends and neighbors who over the years have so generously contributed to this work. My special thanks are due to the members of the Health Hobby Clubs and to the folks trading at the Webster Sq. Pharmacy, whose kind permission to reproduce many of their "family recipes" made this book all the more possible. And for their innumerable suggestions regarding the food and health tips and the therapeutics of the subject matter as herein noted, I am indeed grateful to the authors listed in the bibliography as well as to the listeners of my *Better Health* radio program, the audience at the museum's talks, and the "old-timers" and the farm folk of the New England hinterland. . . .

Introduction

"Economy is in itself a great revenue."—Seneca

Here are presented not only several remedies that were employed by Grandfather Isaiah, a thorough and Thoreauvian herbalist, naturalist and severe teacher; other remedies have been and are still used in medicine, and without difficulty may and should be prepared right in one's own kitchen. . . .

With the exception of salt, sodium bicarbonate, borax and vinegar, all of the items herein listed, yes, even such household commodities as Pepper, the seeds of Pumpkin and Watermelon, Olive and Castor Oil, Corn Starch, I consider *herbs*, and accordingly have recorded their many uses. (And a few other exceptions are the ointment bases of lard and chicken or goose fat, lime water, glycerin, egg and its shells, etc., without which many of the medicinal formulae could not be presented.) To arrive at a proper definition of an herb, one should ever bear in mind that this category includes all such items of vegetable origin that will profitably serve us as medicinal remedies for internal and external purposes, as foods, seasoning agents, as dyes and cosmetics, and even as clothes preservatives. And in the broad category of an herb, we do include the strong spices—Cloves, Ginger, and Mustard, plus their co-conspirators salt and vinegar, all of which, however, are *not* recommended for seasoning; and we include such food-savoring herbs as Anise, Marjoram and Sage; and also portions of shrubs and trees (Barberry, Elder, Sassafras and Linden), house and garden plants, which are generally treated as mere ornamentals (Rose, Marigold, Aloe and Sweet Geranium) and of course the many health-protecting fruits and vegetables which should constitute no less than 80% of our diet. Incidentally, it must be remembered that up to 200 years

9

ago, at which time the word *vegetable* came into being, all of our present-day fruits and vegetables, and plants of an edible nature and of more productive cultivation, were then known as herbs.

🌷   🌷   🌷

The more one studies the therapeutic values of our every-day Nature-all foods, the more will he understand that these foods become the healing agent of most, if not all, organic ailments. Proper selection and balance of organically grown vegetables and fruits, plus proper eating and hygienic habits, become the required fraction of *prevention* of such disorders. Many of the foods, the text will show, have specific healing properties which help to maintain the health of the body, or to prevent sickness; while others are of especial benefit in furthering the recovery from an ailment. Still others exert specific benefits upon the entire blood stream, thus benefiting the liver and bladder and other organs, the nervous system, the bones, etc., the better to maintain the well-being of the body and the individual.

How true it is, as Dr. Harry Finkel has stated in *Diet and Cook Book:*

It is very unfortunate that man has so completely lost himself for thousands of years as to have taken chemicals in an inorganic state in the form of drugs, when these same chemicals could have been obtained in the natural organic state from the plant kingdom. For instance, medical doctors prescribe iron as a tonic for blood when it is found plentifully in Spinach, Apples, Lettuce and Cabbage. Why resort to opium (Ed: and other sedatives) when the Onion and Lettuce possess properties that accomplish the same results? The foods which are most favorable to the reduction of fever and the neutralization of toxins in the body are the acid and sub-acid varieties. These are Limes, Lemons, Grapefruit, Tangerine, Oranges, Pineapple, Plum, Cherries, Apples, Peaches and Pears. Why use dangerous drugs to reduce fever when the acid fruits have a natural tendency to lower the temperature without causing after-effects which are so fearfully dreaded?

These same fruits are of excellent value in breaking up uric acid crystals and aiding greatly in the removal of these toxins from the body. Furthermore, Dr. Finkel has presented the following list of foods to take the place of drugs. Those who are inclined, he wrote, to use special drugs for certain conditions will derive better satisfaction by substituting these foods:

FOODS	DRUGS
Figs	Syrup of Figs
Prunes	Cascarets
Spinach, Cabbage	Iron Tonic
Apples	Castoria
Carrots, Cherries	Blood Tonics
Dried Raspberries, Acid Fruits	Quinine
Wild Cherries, Grapes	Tonics
Tomatoes	Liver Pills
Onions, Lettuce, Celery	Aspirin, Nerve Sedatives
Carrots, Turnips, Radishes	Nerve Tonic
Asparagus, Cauliflower	Kidney Pills

In substance the text will accentuate the positive of self-discipline and frugality, a combination of which should—nay! must—be the unified watch word of every householder. To paraphrase one of Benjamin Franklin's famous and more pertinent sayings: "Take care of the pennies and the dollars will take care of themselves," reminds the writer of Grandfather Isaiah's constant admonitions: "Waste not, want not." It was he, a never-to-be-forgotten shining example of an unswerving conservationist, who first taught us, the three Harris children, the medicinal values of the seeds of Watermelon, Pumpkin and Squash, which we dried and saved for future uses. (In fact, even today several physicians of our city advise the patients to obtain and use such seeds as indicated therein.) "I am also happy to see," he would no doubt add, "that you no longer discard the Radish and Beet tops. The better to prepare them as steamed vegetables or to include them in a soup, and to the soup, will you please add those Carrot tops instead of over-loading the refuse pan? Egg shells you're throwing away? Tsk. Tsk. Excellent fertilizer for your house plants." We would save such everyday items as used Tea leaves (today's Tea bag), Corn Silk and the rinds of Watermelon, which we pickled with native spices as Sassafras, Snakeroot, Wild Allspice and Sweet Flag. It will be later suggested that the rinds of Grapefruit are also to be saved for future use as a "cold breaker"; while those of Orange, Lemon and Tangerine are to be dried and finely ground, later to serve as fruit preserve, seasoning herbs, jelly, or included in an herb tea. Not only did Grandfather guide us along proper gardening habits, for his was the current "organic" method. He would not permit the addition of any chemical as fertilizer or spray: "God provides everything" was one of his favorite expressions; he taught us the many uses of the wonderful herbs of our environs which were of such profitable service to the Harris family, as medicines, foods, material for baskets and clothing, dyes and especially a fishing pole, a whistle and bow and arrows for me. And rarely did Grandfather ever buy his own wine or liquor, for again the Lord had provided him with the almost innate knowledge and skill of preparing his own wines and stronger alcoholic liquors with Wild Grapes, Peaches, Apples, the peelings of Potatoes and of the aforementioned four Citrus friends and a vast array of the ubiquitous and utilitarian herbs—Dandelion, Elder, Burdock and Yarrow, plus a few of the food-savorizers as Sage, Basil, Marjoram et al. Above all, to us grandchildren Grandfather appeared to us as the stalwart standard-bearer of Godliness, Cleanliness and Conservation.

As for eating habits, he advised all adults to eat *one hearty meal a day, usually at suppertime. . . . "Don't,"* he warned, *"eat at all if you're overtired or upset."* Eat many such fruits or vegetables when they are in season. One afflicted with kidney stones should eat such fruits with stones or pits (and it is a well-known fact that these Summer fruits do dissolve out from the body the gravel matter that later may form kidney stones.) And regarding herbs and their remedies, Grandfather's oft-repeated advice amounted to these ever-true tidbits: Use much of the herbs that grow in your immediate environs and remember that "far-fetched is dearly bought." Drink a tea of those herbs twice daily through the year and they will keep your bloodstream clean and toxin-free and your body cool in the summer and warm in the winter. Prepare the body physiologically for the benefits of an herb tea by abstaining from all solid foods for one full day prior to the ingestion of the tea.

Just as his friend the Indian Medicine Man gave thanks

to the Great White Spirit, so Grandfather, too, gave thanks to the Lord for His guidance for his ability to heal, through Nature's produce of wonderful herbs, all who needed healing. Furthermore, it was his policy, as well as of others of his herbalist friends, never to accept money for services rendered, but in payment any handiwork of the patient was accepted as a "fee"—a chair, a basket, or jar of food preserves. I recall especially one token of exchange, a wagonful of the most foul-smelling and very, very dead fish, and drying seaweeds which were to be added to the many composting piles. These piles stood like silent guards, and were spaced ten feet apart around our five acre garden. Never to be forgotten are Grandfather's bits of advice to encourage the householder to stay on a never-ending spree of saving this and saving that, be it foods or herbs or other vegetable or animal matter for some practical economic use as a remedy, or as another addition to the ever-increasing compost piles.

The text will present many household items that are used in present-day medicine and are dispensed by the druggist. The greater number of formulae are simple, the ingredients are on hand and one does not need a college diploma to compound any of the remedies. They are far easier to prepare than meets the skeptic's eye, and take less time than a trip to the corner store for the super-advertised, overpriced proprietaries. As given in this do-it-yourself course, many of the cosmetic recipes, like hand lotion, as well as first-aid remedies for burns, bruises and coughs, are of proven worth, having been prepared for many years and used by the writer and the members of the Health Hobby Clubs.

That a few readers will find cause to doubt the efficacy of certain remedies, there is no doubt; that others, the curious ones, will prefer the druggist's patent remedies and chemical pills, I am sure. (And interestingly enough, the doubters and the curious will remark, as they so very often have to me, "Oh yes, I remember that when we were young, we never had a doctor except on rare occasions. Generally, mother always prepared a cough syrup with Onions and herbs and for a fever gave us a dose or two of hot Sage Tea, etc.") But this book should better qualify one as a kitchen chemist and in time will insure greater and more positive confidence in the ingredients that Nature provides. "For all healing is from God" (Eccl. 38:2). And similarly the homeowner enjoys the satisfied feeling of self-confidence when he landscapes and keeps trim his garden area, when he paints a room, or his garage, when he fixes a minor leak in the plumbing; and self-confidence also comes to the autoist (with or without benefit of AAA or ALA services) who has learned to correct minor troubles of his car. Indeed, the do-it-yourselfer is often rewarded not only by profitable thriftiness but by a more meaningful self-assurance.

Before one ridicules the old-time remedies, let us remember that many of the old-fashioned healing aids are today the newly-found "miracle cures." A news report relating the astonishing effects of some new "wonder" drug has for those wearing the proverbial rose-colored glasses a meaning or interpretation much different from the herbalists'. And in many instances, the modern medical world is turning directly to remedies culled from ancient folklore and the eclectics. A few examples will help give you a clearer picture of just how herbs and vegetables are used today in medicine.

For the past few years, cortisone has held a prominent place in medicine, being used in a variety of diseases, but it was first available in two herbs Wild Yam and Sarsaparilla. Cortisone is comparable to the parillin, one of the active ingredients of our common Sarsaparilla which has been used with excellent success in the treatment of psoriasis and other blood disorders. The natural steroid, parillin, is also found in Yucca and Agave.

A second news line: "Green Hellebore appears to have value in many cases of hypersensitive heart disease." But Hellebore is none other than the famous but highly dangerous veratrum which, my good friend, author Kenneth Roberts of Kennebunkport, Maine, mistook for the mineral-laden and health-fortifying Wild Cabbage. As a result his wife Mrs. Roberts became violently ill. This interesting account is fully discussed in *Eat The Weeds*. However, in medicine, the synthesized ingredient of Hellebore appears as a druggist's item called Veratrine or Veraloid and until recently was extensively prescribed by the physician in cases of hypertension or high blood pressure.

A third item: As a health-hobbyist and naturalist, I have long recommended the eating of steamed or, better, unheated Spinach, and cooked unpearled Buckwheat. These two foods have long been known to be fully packed with a substance needed to insure a strong system of healthy blood vessels. That substance, called rutin, exists also in three garden plants, Rue, Hydrangea and Forsythia. Professor Heber W. Youngken, in his *Textbook of Pharmacognasy*, has written that rutin decreases capillary fragility and reduces the incidence of recurrent hemorrhage associated with a state of increased capillary fragility in diabetic retinitis, pulmonary hemorrhages not caused by tuberculosis. Today, many druggists are filling prescriptions with medicines containing rutin.

Item # 4. Many physicians today prescribe a drug called Dicoumorol for patients ailing with coronary thrombosis, but for decades long before Grandfather's time, an herb which grows right here in New England was used by herbalists for that purpose, as well as for all blood disorders. The herb's name is Yellow Clover, and is closely related to the Common Red Clover. Thus, several years ago, when I read the following report, I was not surprised when some months later, two drug companies came out with a brand new "wonder drug" that according to the advertising, was all that was needed to "cure" the coronaries. I quote the news report: "Announcement of the proceedings of the Mayo Clinic, Rochester, Minnesota, mentions the discovery of a new chemical in Sweet Clover, which was traced to the eating of spoiled Sweet Clover, and led to the discovery. The Wisconsin Experiment Station has completed a seven-year study of clots lodging in the heart or lungs, and in thrombosis. The only practical remedy up to now has been heparin, a liver extract, whose drawback is that it often makes patients ill. Sweet Clover seems to have no such ill effects and the Mayo report states that it may replace heparin in general use. The advantages of this drug are its effectiveness, its prolonged action and its cheapness."

Item #5. We hear so much these days of people suffering with hardening of the arteries; they go to their family doctor and from him receive wise counsel and his suggestions for diet and medication. That is as it should be, but I am of the firm conviction that it is far better to know WHY one's arteries harden and how to take advantage of the oft-maligned and scoffed-at "ounce of prevention" which is the best doctor, since it teaches us the art of self-discipline. And therefore, I believe that the words of the vegetarian, or yes, of the health-minded Jeremiahs, should serve as everlasting warning not to eat highly cholesterolized foods which will eventually clog up the arteries of the blood stream and lead to that dread disease, arteriosclerosis. Furthermore, we should realize that there are, indeed, certain substances that help to prevent that disease, as will all fruits and vegetables, uncooked or raw, wherever possible. And what are these wonder substances that will prevent the hardening of arteries? They are namely, choline and inositol and they are to be found abundantly in green-leaved foods—Dandelion, Spinach and Beet Tops. Please do note that the first substance is called choline and the name of the substance that clogs up the blood arteries is cholesterol which is yielded mainly by fatty meats and processed cheese. Both choline and cholesterol begin with *chol;* the former we need to sustain good health, while the accumulation of the latter in the blood stream increases the danger of poor health.

Item #6. Now let's take another of the so-called "wonder drugs." Folic acid is often prescribed by physicians for disorders of the blood stream. Folic is derived from the Latin word *folia,* a leaf, and folic acid is, therefore, obtained from *all green vegetable matter,* especially from the common Burdock which for centuries has been used as an effective blood purifier.

❦   ❦   ❦

A neighbor of mine, while cleaning out his fireplace, suffered a minor mishap when a small piece of soot or dirt entered his eye. Although he was able to remove the larger particle almost immediately with a Q-tip, there still remained an invisible source of annoyance which still caused great irritation and discomfort. But our friend who today is an herb-minded health enthusiast, had remembered our recent discussion on various herbs and old-time remedies. A moment later, he placed into his troubled eye a whole Flax-seed and in short order, after the jelly of the seed had found its elusive target, friend neighbor was rid of that last particle of dirt and the annoying irritation.

At least two male customers, both nearing the 75 mark

but still "over 40," had related their using Garlic as a cure for bald spots. Their method, unconventional and anti-social as it may appear, consisted of rubbing in the juice of a thin slice of the vegetable-condiment-medicine onto the affected area and allowing the juice to dry. This operation was to be conducted three times a day. In a few weeks, I was told, the bald or balding patches were no more, and had been replaced with an "abundant" crop of hair.

🌷　🌷　🌷

I recall a friend who was advised by her physician to undergo a minor operation for the removal of a large, unsightly mole which, located near her nose, was a source of great annoyance and discomfort. A chance visit with a local "yarb-woman" resulted, strange as it may seem, in the almost complete disappearance of the growth. The remedy? Alternate applications of Castor Oil and the expressed Juice of fresh Cranberries.

The kitchen chemist, ever the true practitioner of conservation, will realize that the ingredents of the remedies indicated thus far and later in the text demand, with very few exceptions, no extra expenditure. These ingredients— Olive Oil, Mustard and Vinegar, etc.—are already at arm's reach in the food cabinet or on the pantry shelf. Furthermore, the kitchener will learn to produce, at a moment's notice, many preparations to effectively heal the ailing, and will generally find these home-made remedies as effective as store-bought patent proprietaries. Take a moment away from your household duties and make this observation: Note the various fruits and vegetables in your refrigerator, the assorted foodstuffs, the herbs and spices on your pantry shelves, the assorted cosmetics in the medicine cabinet, and such chemicals as soap, borax and sodium bicarbonate; then compare them with all the items listed in the text. You will note that with very few exceptions, you have on hand the required ingredients for dozens of remedies, which in most cases, are as effective and even far safer than many store-bought, costly products of similar nature. For the better understanding of matters conversational, which may be dependent upon one's comprehension or interpretation of New England ingenuity or thrift, or a combination of both, let us recall T. T. Munger's remark: "The habit of saving is itself an education; it fosters every virtue, teaches self-denial, cultivates the sense of order, trains to forethought and so broadens the mind."

Further application of the prepare-it-yourself Home Remedy idea is witnessed by its role in Civil Defense and in current calendars' reports concerning "First Aid Information." Civil Defense officials caution the citizenry that if one is "injured in a national disaster, you have to take care of yourself. You may also have to help your injured neighbor as well as your family." Here are a few pertinent examples of Civil Defense remedies: "For eyes irritated by dust, smoke or fumes. Use two drops of Castor Oil in each eye. Apply cold compresses every 20 min, if possible. For shock: Dissolve one teaspoonful of salt and half teaspoonful baking soda in one quart of water. Have patient drink as much as he will." Furthermore, the observant citizen, who practices the "daily theme eye," should observe closely and note well the first aid information on wall-adorning calendars, the Farmer's Almanac, bulletins of insurance companies, and household hints of newspapers and magazines:

1. Antidote for poisoning from Oxalic, Nitric, Hydrochloric, Acetic acids: Give all milk and water that patient can drink—also egg whites.
2. Antidote for alkalies, Lye, Ammonia: Dilute vinegar or lemon juice in water and give to patient.
3. Antidote for Arsenic, Rat Poison: Milk, raw egg, sweet oil, flour and water. Follow with stimulants.
4. Food poisoning (including mushrooms): Give an emetic of mustard and hot water. Follow with milk of magnesia and then with hot coffee. Keep patient quiet and warm.
5. Universal Antidote:

   Powdered burnt toast .... 2 Parts
   Milk of Magnesia .... 1 Part
   Strong Tea .... 1 Part

   Dose: Two teaspoonsful in water
6. Poisoning by wood alcohol, strychnine, bichloride of mercury, carbolic acid: Induce vomiting with mustard

and give stimulants of Tea or Coffee; or a tablespoonful of powdered charcoal mixed in the beverage.

7. Poisoning by Iodine or Moth Balls: Give several whites of eggs and follow with either a mixture of Corn Starch and water or Mustard emetic.

New Poison Antidote: Toast, Tea, Magnesia

Two Duke University doctors have presented what they called a universal antidote for poisons the nature of which is not known. The ingredients: Burned toast, strong tea, milk of magnesia.

The doctors, Jay M. Arena and Grant Taylor of Duke University School of Medicine, presented a scientific exhibit on "Accidental Poisoning in Children" at the annual scientific assembly of the District of Columbia Medical Society.

Doctors who viewed the exhibit told a reporter that such a mixture could well provide a stop gap for people in rural areas isolated from quick medical attention.

The function of the burned toast would be to provide pulverized charcoal to help absorb poisonous materials in the stomach. The tea, containing tannic acid, would help offset an alkaline poison; the milk of magnesia would help offset an acid poison.

Among the home hazards for children are listed:

1. Careless exposure of sugar coated strychnine tablets and other medicines in the home cabinets within reach of youngsters and similar exposure of sleeping tablets on bedside tables.

2. Allowing babies to play in rooms treated with anti-roach poisons or in attics where they might eat moth balls.

They said children could get aniline dye poisoning from eating red and orange waxed crayons.   *News Report.*

How to Prevent Accidental Poisoning in Your Home

Keep all drugs, poisonous substances, and household chemicals out of the reach of children and under lock and key if necessary.

Store non-edible products in their original containers; do not transfer them to unlabeled containers.

When medicines are discarded, destroy them. Do not throw them where they might be reached by children or pets.

When giving flavored and/or brightly colored medicine to children, always refer to it as a medicine—NOT AS CANDY.

Do not take or give medicine in the dark.

Read labels before using chemical products.

Florida Health Notes.

The dangers of certain chemicals like salt, sodium bicarbonate, mineral oil have been briefly discussed if only to show—in such a small space so allotted—the great harm that comes from the continual ingestion of chemical drugs and of poisonous chemicals. Furthermore, I have indicated in many instances that the everyday use of conventional seasoning agents such as salt and vinegar (white), spices of Clove, Cinnamon, Ginger and Mustard and other mischief makers, should be used at an extreme minimum or, better, not at all; that the conventional table-use of such maldoers will bring on more quickly the conventional organic disorders and that they should be replaced by the culinary seasoners —Basil, Marjoram and Sage—for your better health.

Much of the material herein presented has been taken from *The Medicine of Our Foods* (of which the completed manuscript was lost in its entirety in the dreadful flood of August 1955) and will in most instances indicate: 1. The major constituents of foods and their relative percentages. 2. How to prepare these foods for table use and with which other foods to combine them for better digestion and assimilation. 3. A new concept in cooking: Eat as much of your foods that can be eaten uncooked (unheated and unfired); if the heavier root vegetables need heating, *steam* these but only a very few minutes and in very little water and only long enough that they may be then chewed. Remember, too, that certain foods like Spinach and Rhubarb and other oxalic acid bearers, if prepared in the conventional manner, i.e. boiled in hot water, will yield the free oxalic acid which in time leeches out and therefore eliminates the much needed blood-fortifying calcium from the blood stream.

The Wonder Drugs of yesterday are the Blunder Drugs of today.

Kitchen Medicines

ALLSPICE

These are the unripe fruits of a beautiful evergreen tree that is indigenous to the West Indies and South America. Commonly known as Pimentos, they possess a strong clovelike taste and pronounced aromatic odor and are popular among cooks as a condiment for seasoning meats, fish, soups and stews. As a medicinal, they have long been recommended as an aromatic stomachic for habitual colics.

Allspice Water: Boil ½ to ¾ teaspoonful of bruised or ground fruits in a pint of hot water for 10 minutes. Strain and drink a tablespoonful (plain or diluted with warm water to suit the taste) as required. This decoction may be used as a carminative for flatulence, colic, etc.

Compound Spice Wine: A heaping teaspoonful each of All-Spice, Cinnamon and Clove, all powdered, are mixed into a pint of warm wine. The utensil is covered until cool, then stirred and strained. Two teaspoonsful make a dose and are used as an aromatic and carminative.

❦   ❦   ❦

"We put drugs, about which we know little, into our bodies, about which we know less, to cure diseases, about which we know nothing at all."   *William Osler, M.D.*

❦   ❦   ❦

SWEET ALMOND

It was Martius, the famed botanist, who suggested that the name Almond had its derivation in the Hebrew *shakad,* "be wakeful," "keep guard." The English name, Almond, is derived from the Latin *amandula,* a corruption of *amygdala.*

The nut is one of the richest sources of protein, high in vitamins A and B and in minerals calcium, phosphorus, magnesium and potassium. It is best combined with raw, non-starchy vegetables and acid fruits. With Almonds as with all other nuts, eat *no* starches, sugars or other forms of protein. A well rounded meal may consist of a large salad of fresh vegetables and a half cup of Almonds, well chewed.

Almond meal or powder is a by-product in the manufacture of Almond oil and is largely used as a detergent powder for local irritations of the skin. The expressed oil, states *The United States Dispensatory,* has the advantage of comparative tastelessness and freedom from odor and lack of tendency to become gummy, and because of its known emollient properties, is widely used as an emollient for chapped hands and other inflamed conditions of the skin.

Dr. William Meyrick said that the oil of Almonds was much employed in his times, in tickling cough and habitual costiveness, with success. And the nuts themselves, he advised, were to be blanched and beaten into an emulsion with Barley Water, which was of great use in the stone, gravel, strangury and other disorders of the kidneys, bladder and biliary (gall bladder) ducts.

Emulsion of Almond (U.S.P.IX.) ("Milk of Almond"): Sweet Almond (nuts), 2 oz., blanched; Powered Acacia, 2½ tsp.; Brown Sugar, 1 ounce, or 2 oz. Honey. Grind the almonds, beat them with the other 2 ingredients until thoroughly mixed. Add 1½ pints of water, very gradually and stir until a uniform mixture results. Strain and add enough water to make a quart. The emulsion should be freshly prepared.

This is an excellent preparation for use as a demulcent nutritive and emollient where solid foods cannot be taken.

Almond Powder: Mix together 4 oz. each of Almond meal and Rice flour and ½ ounce of Orris root powder. The powder is used as a demulcent to soothe skin irritations.

Almond Powder (meal) Cleanser: Mix well 2 ounces of Almond powder (meal), 1 ounce of Kaolin, a half teaspoonful of Borax and then add a few drops of perfume. Use as a soap substitute for inflammations of the skin.

❦   ❦   ❦

ALOE

There are many uses for this ornamental house plant which
requires little care and very little water. The gummy exudation of the leaves yields the virtues and may be used alone
or mixed with other ingredients. For chapped or rough hands
and insect bites, the freshly expressed juice is applied directly,
and similarly in the case of sunburn or scald. For the latter
conditions a strong warm decoction of pekoe tea is prepared,
to which Irish Moss is added to form a jelly. To this mixture
the clear gummy juice of the Aloe is added. This preparation
has been found to be the most soothing and healing. The gum
yields a substance called aloin, which is used extensively in
medicine as a tonic laxative and purgative in habitual constipation. It has been reported to the writer that the laxative
action may be obtained from the leaf by immersing a portion
of cut leaf in tap water for 10-15 minutes, straining and
drinking the filtrate at night a half hour before retiring and
again in the morning if necessary.

Other uses include: The pulp and juice of the fresh leaf
to increase the rate of healing of X-ray burns; the extracted
juice of the Aloes as a varnish to preserve wood from
worms and white ants; the juice applied to the skins of man
or beast as an insect repellent; mixed with turpentine, white
lead, and tallow, to preserve a ship's bottom from the
ravages of worms and the adhesion of barnacles.

Alvagel (a product of Miami, Florida): Contains not less
than 55% of the *Aloe Vera* fresh leaf gel in a base of cho
lesterolized petrolatum. For minor skin abrasions, minor cuts,
minor sunburn and minor burns.

A-Gic (New York City, N.Y.), a product consisting of a
78% concentration of Aloe pulp, has long been employed by
physicians and clinics in the treatment and relief of burns,
etc.

"Economy is half the battle in life; it is not so hard to earn
money, as to spend it well."   *Charles H. Spurgeon.*

ANISE

Anise seeds are generally used as a substitute for Caraway

to flavor pastries and cookies; and with or without powdered Cinnamon to season Apple preparations—sauce, stew, pies and salads. A sprinkle of the seeds over these foods will act as the grain of prevention by helping to overcome faulty digestion.

The therapeutic properties of the aromatic seeds should not be overlooked. They act as a soothing carminative. Children who are troubled with colic or flatulence should drink, during and after meals, a cup of warm infusion of the seeds, with results almost guaranteed (see below). And Anise seeds also help to prevent the griping of laxatives (Cascara pills or Senna Leaves), and if the habitual laxative-taker will drink more frequently herbal teas of Anise and like aromatic herbs, the greater will be the opportunity to free himself from this unhealthy and dangerous habit of laxative taking.

The seeds should enter into home-made cough syrups and lozenges and its medicinal virtues are best demonstrated as an invaluable aid to prevent and eliminate catarrhal conditions of the alimentary and bronchial passages. Thus the druggist's prescription items of Spirits of Anise, Spirits of Anisated Ammonia, and Anise Water. During the "Virus X" epidemic of 1950's winter, the following prescription was filled at our Pharmacy: Essence of Anise (Spirit)—1 oz. Sig: Dose: 15 drops in a quart of steaming water for inhalation. . . . Dr. W. (This inhalation helped a severe case of laryngitis.)

Cough Remedy: In a cup of hot water, steep a half-teaspoonful each of the seeds and Thyme. When cool, stir and strain. Add a teaspoonful of honey. Sip slowly every ½-1 hour, two tablespoonsful. This syrup is especially adapted for young children and infants.

Cough Remedy for Adults: Simmer one teaspoonful each of Horehound, Thyme, Anise and Licorice (or Hollyhock Root) in a pint of hot water for 10 minutes. Stir and strain. Dissolve a cup of brown sugar or honey in the liquid and allow to cool. Strain into a clean bottle and cover. Dose: A tablespoonful sipped slowly every hour or as needed to relieve the irritation due to cough or cold.

The seeds are ingredients in other remedies for cough syrup and lozenges to be found under Thyme. (See Sugar.)

Sluggish Liver: Mix 2 ounces of Dandelion leaves with ½

ounce each of Anise, Fennel and Flax-seed. Simmer for 15 minutes ⅓ of the mixture in a pint of hot water, cover, and let stand half hour. Stir and strain. The dose is a cupful morning and night.

Colic Remedy: Mix well ¼ teaspoonful each of Anise, Fennel, Ground Mint and Catnip in a cup of hot water and cover 10 min. Stir and strain. For the adults and children, the dose is the entire cupful sipped slowly. For infants, restrain through absorbent cotton into a 4-ounce nursing bottle, so that the infusion may be taken via the nipple; or baby may prefer teaspoonful doses.

Antacid (Colic): Use ¼ teaspoonful each of Anise, Fennel, Caraway and Dill and prepare as directed under *Colic Remedy.* This preparation was known to druggists as Compound Anise Water and is especially useful in overcoming colic in infants and the aged. For the dose, see the previous remedy.

Anise Water: Prepare an infusion by steeping 2 teaspoonsful in a pint of hot water. Cover 10 minutes and strain. Dose: A tablespoonful sipped slowly as needed.

Syrup of Anise: Dissolve 3½ ounces of brown sugar in 4 ounces of cold Anise Water. Use as a colic or cough remedy. Dose: A teaspoonful as needed, sipped slowly.

🌷   🌷   🌷

APPLES

The apple is a delicious and nutritious fruit and alkaline in reaction when eaten uncooked ("raw") and unpeeled. It is rich in Vitamins C, B and G and minerals potassium, iron, sodium and magnesium, and these elements help to greatly *strengthen the blood stream.* Malic and tartaric acids are also contained in the fruits and are of great value to persons held to sedentary habits which may account for possible disturbances of the digestion and liver. Apples are best combined with Pears, Grapes, Peaches and other such fruits, although a second choice of Bananas, Figs, and Dates may also be considered. Do not eat Apples with acid fruits (Oranges, Lemons, etc.), Bread, Cereal, and Nuts.

One authority states, "In countries where unsweetened cider is used as a beverage, (kidney) stone or calculus is unknown," and that not a single case of kidney stone had been met with during forty years in Normandy, France.

Apples Inhibit Tooth Decay

Some nice news in the Medical Press for apple lovers—an apple a day can keep the dentist away too. Though there was much speculation on the role apples could play in cleansing the teeth of decay-causing nests of refined carbohydrates, no one ever did much to prove it. Two British doctors, Slack and Martin, set about experimenting along these lines and had gratifying results. Two groups of children were selected at random, representing various ages to 15 years. One group ate a thin slice or two of raw apple after each meal or snack, while the others did not. It was found that the low acidity of the apples stimulated a rare salivary flow. The apple particles sweeping over the teeth with the increased saliva removed debris and stimulated gum tissues. The authors wrote that the gum condition of the children eating apples was significantly better than the other group, and the effect on reducing caries was also encouraging. They felt that a larger, more controlled study of the effect of apples on the inhibition of dental caries is in order. We agree. Anything which will call attention to the effectiveness of this natural food should be promoted by all who have become disgusted with the false claims of modern toothpastes.   From *Prevention*.

An Apple a Day

Now you can reach for an apple instead of a tranquilizer. A three year check on the effects of apple eating on the general health of students at Michigan State University indicates that students who eat two apples a day have fewer tensions, headaches, and emotional upsets than those who eat none, by a 12 to 1 ratio. Furthermore, says Harold Tukey, head of the department of horticulture, preliminary results show that those who eat apples have fewer skin diseases, arthritic ailments and upper respiratory difficulties.   *News Report*.

The active medicinal principle of this fruit is Pectin, one of two therapeutic ingredients of the druggist's Kao-Pectate, which is usually used for the usual summer complaints of children. The Kao portion is Kaolin, a form of white porcelain or china clay and somewhat similar to Fuller's Earth.

The Pectin (Pectate) is obtained from the dilute acid extract of the inner portion of the rinds or from Apple pomace. It is recognized as an "official" drug and is used extensively in the pharmaceutical and cosmetic industries. It is also used as an emulsifying and gelling agent and enters into such products as pastes for external application, hair pomades, dentifrices, etc.

The Upjohn Company, makers of Kaopectate, state that Apple Pectin supplements the protective coating action of the Kaolin, by virtue of its action as an absorbent and demulcent, aiding detoxification by supplying galacturonic acid necessary for the elimination of certain noxious substances. Pectin helps to prevent putrefaction of protein matter in the alimentary canal.

An old time remedy for diarrhea, still in use today, is to simmer apple parings in boiled milk, a half cupful being drunk warm every hour until relieved.

Here are a few typical examples of the Apple's uses, associated with the folklore and superstition in which the fruit abounds. In Germany, the fruit is mixed with Saffron petals for use against jaundice. And in Silesia, the Apple is scraped from the top to cure summer complaints (diarrhea) and from the bottom to cure costiveness. Many an Italian of the past generation will warn you, if you are a singer:

> "Pome, pere ed noce
> Guastano la voce,"

"Apples, Pears and Nuts spoil the voice."

In certain parts of Europe, a sure sign of disaster or death is the blooming of the Apple tree after the fruit is ripe. Want to get rid of your wart? In Devonshire, England, it was the custom to cut an Apple in two, rub each half over the wart, tie them together again, and bury them near a cemetery.

Cider in Gout and Rheumatism

"Cider has long been held to be an excellent beverage for persons of a gouty or rheumatic constitution. It was noticed long ago, that in the cider-drinking districts, stone and gravel are relatively uncommon. There has been considerable discussion about the explanation, but the fact has not been controverted by those medical men most familiar with the cider-drinking regions of England. It is quite possible that the slight acidity in cider acts as an intestinal germicide or inhibitant, thus restraining the excessive growth of the putrefactive organisms always present in an attack of gout. Further, malic acid is a decided diuretic, so that its action on the kidneys may promote urinary excretion and hence the elimination of uric acid."   *Meyer's Almanac.*

Appella is a product of the Winthrop Laboratories and consists of Apple powder with 5% of Kaolin. The label reads: "Appella contains fruit sugars, salts, organic acids and other valuable constituents of the apple in powder form. Valuable in all conditions in which pectin, uronic acids and fruit carbohydrates are indicated. . . . Indicated for simple diarrhea associated with dietary disturbances and as a supplement to infant feeding."

🌷   🌷   🌷

ARTICHOKE

The receptacle and bases of the scaled flower-heads are eaten as a vegetable. They are best prepared when steamed only a few minutes, long enough to be softened and to be chewed properly, and quickly to preserve the nutrients.

It has long been employed as a medicine. Dr. Meyrick, in 1740, had stated that "the juice of the leaves, or a strong decoction of the roots is powerfully diuretic, and of great efficacy in the jaundice and dropsy, which will frequently yield to this medicine without any other assistance but the divine blessing." To which one authority adds that the very bitter leaves of artichokes were at one time thought to be diuretic and used in dropsies and rheumatism.

Diuretic Remedy: Two tablespoonfuls (one each) of dried and finely cut leaves of Artichoke and Asparagus are boiled in a pint of hot water for 5 minutes, allowed to cool and strained. A half cupful is drunk every 3 to 4 hours, care being taken to abstain from eating for at least 2 hours before each dose.

ASPARAGUS

This food is best prepared by being steamed for 3 or 4 minutes in as little water as possible. Thus the nutrients are not dissipated nor their values lost. 1. Asparagus contains an appreciably high percentage of vitamins A and C; 2. Minerals of calcium, phosphorus, sodium, chlorine, sulfur and potassium; 3. A large amount of a therapeutically active substance called asparagine which is of great benefit in cases of kidney disfunction. (This principle is found also in the roots of Marshmallow Herb).

Asparagus is strongly diuretic in action and to a lesser degree, deobstruent and aperient. Dr. R. D. Pope says that "since the juice of this vegetable helps the breaking up of oxalic acid crystals in the kidneys and throughout the muscular system, it is good for rheumatism, neuritis, etc. Rheumatism results from the end products of the digestion of meat and meat products, generating excessive amount of urea (uric acid)."

Asparagus Root is mentioned in *The Pharmaceutical Recipe Book* as an ingredient in "Five Roots Tea," the other herbs being the roots of Celery, Fennel, Parsley, and Butcher's Broom, all in equal parts. The Tea is prepared by simmering 2 teaspoonsful in 10 ounces of boiling water for 5 minutes. When cool, the mixture is stirred, strained and drunk. Our Diuretic Pill, manufactured by Hance Bros. and White of Philadelphia, Pa., contains Asparagus, Corn Silk, Oil of Juniper, Licorice, and *uva ursi* (Bearberry).

Decoction of Asparagus:
1. Boil one ounce of the dried cut roots in 2 pints of hot water, boil 10 minutes and allow to cool. Stir, strain and drink one such cupful 4 times a day. This preparation has been used in dropsy.
2. Boil one ounce in a pint of water *(The Dispensatory)* and prepare as in #1.
3. Simmer a heaping tablespoonful of cut roots in a pint of hot water for a half hour. Take a tablespoonful of resultant liquid every 2 hours.

❦   ❦   ❦

BANANA

Doctors Report Bananas Cure Abdominal Ill

A dangerous abdominal disease that strikes mostly young children and often causes death can now be diagnosed and cured by a diet featuring bananas, two physicians reported. The ailment is known in medical circles as celiac disease. Diarrhea and failure to gain weight are the chief symptoms.

The report of a cure by proper diet was published by Drs. Sidney V. and Merrill P. Haas of the Vanderbilt clinic in the magazine *Postgraduate Medicine*. It is the first time a cure has been reported.

The physicians said they based their findings on a study of 603 cases, most of whom were children. In reviewing the limited research into causes and cure of the disease, the doctors said, celiac disease causes altered intestinal function. "From this altered intestinal function may come varying degrees of disturbance of nutrition depending upon the duration and severity of the condition and upon the diet," they said. Dr. Haas said the disease may occur at any age, although it is encountered most commonly among children under six. They said the condition can be improved and eventually cured through a diet.

Some patients, they said, ate as many as 10 bananas a day. But in prescribing the diet, the physicians said, it is more important to list what can not be fed. They said: "Any cereal grain is strictly and absolutely forbidden, including corn, wheat, rye or rice in any form, whether as bread, cake, toast, crackers or breakfast cereals. Potato is prohibited. Sugar is forbidden as sweetening or in the form of candy, pastries, breads, etc., as well as dextrins, such as are found in corn syrups and other lollypops. Milk is not allowed."

Diagnosis of the disease, the doctors said, can be made simply by feeding one of the forbidden items to the suspected case after the prescribed diet has been put into effect. If the symptoms return after improvement has been made, the diagnosis is confirmed, the doctors said. By observing the diet, most cases begin to improve immediately. And when cure is obtained there should be no relapse.   *News Report.*

They Call Him The Banana Kid

During the past 3½ years, 5 year old Willard Hadley of

Seattle has eaten three tons of bananas—more than 17,000 of them. And he still likes them! He was stricken with celiac disease when he was 1½ years old, and bananas were part of his necessary diet. Now he's cured, but he still thinks the tropical fruit has great appeal. *News Report.*

This delicious food is best eaten when the skin darkens and is speckled with small dark spots. It is an excellent source of Vitamins A, B, G, and Riboflavin and of minerals, potassium, sodium and chlorine. It may be eaten with non-starchy vegetables, other fruits but not with acid fruits, such as Oranges or Tangerines, etc., and never with starches or proteins.

> A banana is the world's most portable breakfast,
> On what do I this bold, broad statement base?
> It is filling, needs no cooking, is nutritious,
> And it has its own bright yellow carrying case!

BARLEY

The pearled cereal has proven to be one of the mildest and least irritating of that type of food and has been much used as a nutritive and demulcent drink in cases of bowel diseases, debilitated conditions of the system and catarrhal affections. And too, a demulcent drink is indicated in febrile and inflammatory diseases where solid foods cannot be taken. Barley water is prepared by boiling two ounces of the cereal in two quarts of hot water down to about one quart or so, and carefully straining. This mucilagenous drink has been much employed, we are informed, "from the time of Hippocrates to the present. It is especially used in infant feeding, as it seems to prevent the formation of large milk curds by its colloidal character."

The Barley decoction was much used in the mid 1700's and when Dr. Meyrick advised his patients to take much of this "most elegant grateful beverage, which is extremely useful in the·gravel, stone, strangury, and the heat of urine; likewise in fevers of the ardent kind, and other acute disorders where cooling and diluting are necessary."

From malted Barley, there has been extracted, one authority states, a substance known as Hordenine, which has been used "in the treatment of various forms of diarrhea and dysentery and in gastric hyper-secretion." The writer finds that Hordenine has a powerful effect in overcoming bronchial spasm and suggests its use in asthma. It has been chiefly used in intestinal disorders and as a cardiac tonic.

1. *Decoction of Barley.* The ingredients are 2 ounces of Barley and 3½ pints of water. Boil the Barley in 8 ounces of water for a few minutes, drain off this water, add the remainder in a boiling state and boil down to one-half and strain. The preparation is employed as a nutritive and demulcent drink in febrile and inflammatory diseases.

2. *Compound Decoction of Barley:* The ingredients are 2 pints of Decoction of Barley, 2½ ounces of sliced Figs, ½ ounce cut Licorice root, 2½ ounces of Raisins and one pint of water. Mix and boil down to 2 pints, and strain. (From the *London Pharmacopoeia*). This is a demulcent, nutritive and somewhat laxative drink.

3. (A). *Prepared Barley Meal:* Tie it (any amount) in a linen cloth and boil it for 12 hours, then let it cool, remove the outer crust and pulverize the center. When boiled in milk, this has been considered to be of good service in bowel disorders.

(B). *Prepared Barley Meal:* 12 ounces Barley Meal, 4 ounces of sugar and ½ teaspoonful of powdered Cinnamon are mixed with a small amount of whole wheat flour and baked into small cakes. In the early part of the century, this spiced Barley Cake was much in vogue as a "tonic in debilitated conditions of the systems."

Pearled Barley is used as the "medicine"; only the unpearled food can be considered as the proper article of diet, for in its untampered state, it contains its optimum of vitamin B complex factors and minerals calcium, magnesium, phosphorus, potassium and sodium. Barley is best eaten with vegetables.

BASIL

Basil is popularly employed in cookery as a seasoning for soups, stews, meats and egg and cheese dishes. It should be used fresh in vegetable salads, and alone or with Garlic may be vinegared. It is easily grown from seeds sown directly into the garden in late May. The herb, an annual, is a prodigious grower and will yield several cuttings.

I have noted that some folks afflicted with an overdose of rheumatic pains have found in Basil not a sure cure but at least a means of temporarily allaying their suffering. A warm infusion of the leaves of curly Basil is said to be a popular remedy for rheumatism in Japan, while the Sacred Basil is used similarly in India. They, like so many non-rheumatics, have enjoyed the satisfying, aromatic soups of the tender young leaves prepared Spinach style, and after their meals, a warm tea of Basil, Catnip or Peppermint.

Of each herb, infuse ⅓ teaspoonful in a cup of hot water for five minutes. Stir, strain, sip slowly one such cupful 4-5 times a day. Basil serves also as a mild tonic for nervous disorders and helps to offset stomach catarrh. To the preceding recipe, you may add ⅓ teaspoonful of Sage and prepare as directed.

Have a headache and need a simple remedy to be applied as a compress? It is easily prepared. Infuse a teaspoonful of dried, ground Basil in a cup of hot water for 8 to 10 minutes and strain. When the liquid is cool, add 2 tablespoonsful of Witch Hazel extract, previously chilled. Apply the solution as a compress to the forehead and temples. (Of course, the enterprising herbalist would use the leaves and twigs of Witch Hazel, collected in Fall, to prepare his own extract).

❦   ❦   ❦

BEANS

The kidney Bean, *Phaseolus Vulgaris,* was at one time held in high repute as a good diuretic, "to cleanse the kidneys and ureters of gravel and fabulous concretions," while one medical authority held the various parts of the garden Bean, *Vicia Faba,* in high esteem as medicinal agents. Said he: "The distilled water of Bean flowers is in great request as a cosmetic, and is said to soften the skin, and free it from sunburning, spots, pimples and freckles, etc. . . . Many people distil a water from the pods (Ed: A simple decoction may also be used), which is of a carminative nature, and being destitute of heat and acrimony, is an excellent medicine for young children who are troubled with griping pains in the stomach and bowels. . . . The leaves beaten into a poultice with cream, cool and repel inflammatory tumors, and heal burns and scalds. . . . A poultice made with bean-meal, is good to remove inflammation arising from wounds and bruises. . . . Country people sometimes make use of the juice of the leaves to take away warts."

🌷   🌷   🌷

I solemnly swear I will eat to live, not live to eat.
I will eat sensibly, carefully.
I will get weighed every day.
I will keep a chart, recording what I have eaten and at what time.
I will read one new book every month, one that will give me an inspiring viewpoint on life.
I will make a serious effort to understand myself, weighing my findings honestly, accenting my good points, and minimizing or overcoming my faults.
I will do something different at least one day each week.
I will make at least one new friend or acquaintance each month.
And finally, I will cultivate my sense of awareness, studying other people, how they affect me and why, and how I affect them, study their qualities and mind.

Ruth Douglas, *Fatties Anonymous.*

🌷   🌷   🌷

BEET

This food may be grated and added to a vegetable salad and so eaten uncooked. If it must be cooked, it should be steamed but a few minutes, without removing the skin and in as little water as possible. And *eat the greens for they are an important article of food.* Beets are best combined with non-starchy vegetables. Not only are vitamins A, B, C, and G contained in the Beet; there are these blood building minerals calcium, chloride, phosphorus, potassium, silicon, sodium and sulfur. It is important to note that sodium is in proper proportion to calcium, i.e. 10 to 1, thus insuring the desired solubility of the latter.

The potassium content of 20%, Dr. R. D. Pope tells us, "furnishes the general nourishment for all the physiological functions of the body, while the 8% content of chlorine furnishes a splendid organic cleanser of the liver, kidneys and gall bladder, also stimulating the activity of the lymph throughout the body." Dr. Pope also believes that "the iron in red beets, although not of a high content," is nevertheless of a quality that furnishes excellent food for the red corpuscles of the blood.

In the days of George Washington, the physicians recommended the juice of the fresh white roots as "an excellent remedy for the headache, and that species of toothache in which the whole jaw and side of the face is affected."

Another Home Remedy: Back in the 16th century, when doctors were few and far between and medical science was in its infancy, Beet juice was used in treating earaches. Three or four drops were supposed to be put in the ailing ear. And Dr. Wood had written that the roots of the red Beet were, "very efficacious in gravel and a number of urinary complaints as catarrh of the bladder, inflammation of the kidneys, etc."

🌷   🌷   🌷

COMPOUND TINCTURE OF BENZOIN

The average householder buys from the druggist a one or two ounce bottle of Compound Tincture of Benzoin (Co. Tr. Benzoin), which is intended to be used generally as a steam inhalation. For this purpose, a teaspoonful of the tincture is placed in a pint of hot water and the vapors are inhaled, and this procedure is indicated in the early stages of acute bronchitis or whooping cough. Often do medical doctors prescribe the tincture for its stimulating expectorant value for the relief of chronic bronchitis. The householder in need of a similar remedy for laryngitis or bronchitis may prepare a syrup by slowly and thoroughly mixing a teaspoonful in 4 ounces of favorite cough syrup, which for best results, should be sipped slowly.

However, the kitchen chemist will find in Co. Tr. Benzoin a most reliable remedy for further applications: For chapped hands, a half teaspoonful may be incorporated in 8 ounces of either a standard hand lotion or in one described under Irish

Moss or Cucumber. As a local application to minor wounds
and indolent ulcers, it may be either mixed in equal portions
of unsalted lard and lanolin (½ teaspoonful to 1 ounce ointment or base), or it may be applied as is tincture of iodine,
thinly and as often as every hour. In this vulnerary respect, its
antiseptic and protective properties are of inestimable value.

❦   ❦   ❦

BLACKBERRY

As the fruits ripen, they lose their astringency, i.e., the
tannic acid content becomes safely lodged in the root, for
which reason the unripe berries and root have been used since
Biblical days as an astringent for dysentery, and a gargle for
sore throat.

However, the ripe sweet fruits are to be used as are other
sub-acid fruits, Raspberry, Elderberry, etc. Although best eaten
uncooked with other fruits as Banana and Peach, and dairy
products, they too, are excellent material for jam, jelly and
conserve. Yes, Blackberries are alkaline in reaction.

According to Meyrick, the unripe berries were more astringent than any other part and were used to good purpose "in
all manner of fluxes and hemorrhages." Formerly the leaves
were decocted and with a little honey added the decoction
was used as a gargle for thrush and other irritations of the
throat. A tea of the flowers was also considered diuretic and
anti-lithic.

The Fall-collected roots of this common herb have long
been used as an astringent remedy for diarrhea and dysentery.
For this purpose one ounce or 2 tablespoonsful of the roots,
finely ground, are boiled in 1½ pints of hot water down to a
pint and allowed to cool. The dose is one or two ounces, 3-4
times a day as required.

Where a less bitter remedy is indicated for an infant or
child, the fresh fruits may be used by simmering for 10 minutes half a cupful of the expressed juice with one of brown
sugar. Strain and allow to cool. This syrup must be freshly
prepared when needed and stored in the refrigerator. That is
why we recommend that any excess of fruits of the Summer
collection be *dehydrated*, to be used when needed.

Blackberry Cordial: Boil for 10 minutes in a pint of hot

water a cupful of the ripe fruits, 2 cupsful of sugar, 2 or 3 Cloves and 2 small pieces of Cinnamon. Allow to cool, stir and strain. To the strained liquid, add an equal amount of port wine. The dose is a tablespoonful in warm water as needed to check the diarrhea or similar complaint.

❦ ❦ ❦

BLUEBERRY

Blueberries may well boast of many virtues: To be sure they offer a most satisfying Summer dessert and represent a free-for-the-asking product of Nature's own vast garden. The leaves and twigs possess medicinal properties. An abnormally functioning kidney tract is soon remedied by prepared infusions. Moreover, it is little realized that the leaves yield myrtillin, a substance which is now known to reduce blood sugar as does insulin. The fruits tend to act as a new-fashioned blood purifier, such action depending upon the blood fortifying minerals as calcium, iron, and phosphorus and one other, equally as important as these three, namely manganese. The latter acts as a catalyzing agent on behalf of the blood stream; that is, it helps to conduct into the blood stream the Blueberry's calcium, iron and phosphorus content, and thus enhance the assimilation of these minerals. (See under Thyme for "Blood Cleanser" formula.)

Preparation. The fresh fruits are well reputed for their food values, best eaten uncooked and without sugar. They are also preserved and included in pies and pastries.

Jellies are best made when prepared with sour apple. Any excess of the berries should be sun-dried (or attic-dried) and later in the Fall may be included in puddings and cakes. Allow 10-12 days for complete drying and the berries will resist decay or mold.

The Dispensatory states under myrtillin, "this name has been applied to a substance of unknown composition which was originally obtained from *Vaccinium Myrtillus*. . . . The Blueberry leaf has been used as a folk remedy in the treatment of diabetes for many years. Allen reports favorable effects in a number of cases of diabetes."

To prepare an anti-diabetes tisane for the non-user of insulin, drugs, etc., steep a teaspoonful of the cut dried leaves in a cup of hot water. Drink one such cupful four times a day. Self-discipline and strict adherence to an all-natural diet are far more important than remedies and "cures." With equal parts of Parsley and Strawberry leaves, Blueberry enters into a kidney remedy prepared as the tisane previously mentioned.

🌱　　🌱　　🌱

BORAX

This chemical is the druggist's Sodium Borate and for all purposes must be marked U.S.P. (United States Pharmacopœia). Except as a gargle or mouth wash, Borax must not be taken internally, i.e., swallowed. *The United States Dispensatory* states that "in sufficient amounts it exerts a depressing influence upon the heart as well as upon the spinal centers, and a number of instances of poisoning from it have been reported. The symptoms have varied somewhat but in most, if not all, cases there have been great depression of spirits, fall of bodily temperature, a very feeble pulse—rapid or slow —and an erythematous eruption accompanied with much swelling of the parts, and especially affecting the lower extremities, and followed by exfoliation; nausea, violent vomiting and hiccough have been present in some cases. The mind usually remains clear until late in the poisoning, but death has been preceded by coma with disturbances of the respiration, and involuntary discharges."

Borax has long been used in medicine as a wash for external ulcers and abscesses, for which purpose a solution is prepared in strength of one part of Borax to 14 of water. Borax is sometimes added to soaps to serve as a detergent ingredient.

Its use as an ant-powder is mentioned under Red Pepper, which see.

Almond Meal and Borax Cleanser: The ingredients are 2 ounces of Almond Meal, 1 ounce of Kaolin and a half teaspoonful of Borax. These are mixed together and used as a cleansing agent where soap is not desired.

Glycerite of Borax: In 3 ounces of Glycerine, slightly warmed, dissolve ½ ounce of Borax. Use as a swab for thrush of infants and sore throat of children.

Gargle: Mix 2 teaspoonsful Borax and 1 ounce Honey in 8 ounces of hot water. Use warm for sore throat and thrush.

Borax Honey: Stir well a level teaspoonful of Borax in an ounce of warmed Honey. This is often prescribed by our local physicians as an application for aphtha and thrush of children.

Vinegar of Borax: Warm 2 ounces of Malt or Cider Vinegar and in it dissolve a teaspoonful of Borax. This is an old-time remedy for ringworm of the scalp.

Ointment of Borax: Incorporate a level teaspoonful in an ounce of butter or lard. Apply to scaly eruptions of the skin.

To remove tea and cocoa stains, soak the article in a solution of borax and water.

❦   ❦   ❦

TWO WAY DIET—TRIET

What you DON'T put in your face,
CAN'T add pounds some other place.
Second Helpings CAN'T add weight,
IF you leave them on the plate.
What you DON'T put in your mind,
Won't be hard to leave behind.

Don Blanding

❦   ❦   ❦

BRAN

In the past few years, bran has been advertised as a laxative food. Such action, says *The Dispensatory,* "is probably mechanical consisting in the irritation produced upon the mucous membrane of the bowels by its coarse particles. In cases of irritability of the colon, it may do much harm." Forewarned is forearmed. The taking of bran in any form, for whatever purpose, is not recommended because of possible irritations.

❦   ❦   ❦

BREAD

Bread, in its various forms, has long been employed as a medicinal agent for diverse conditions. The wheat flour was at one time used as a desiccant dusting powder, but as *The Dispensatory* tells us, "has been completely replaced by powdered starch." A poultice is often made by boiling bread with milk. The effects of this poultice are similar to those of a Flax-seed poultice although it does not hold the heat so well.

Cataplasma Panis (Bread Poultice) is still retained in the *Pharmaceutical Recipe Book* (3rd Ed.), if only as a gentle reminder that many of our everyday foods frequently may serve two-fold, as a nutritive and as a healing remedy. The poultice is prepared by immersing bread or the crumbs in boiling water for 5 minutes, then straining off the water and spreading the mass over the affected area. To prepare a poultice or cataplasm of the crumbs, moisten them with enough warm milk and freshly roasted chopped onion and apply.

Bread crumbs were formerly used by the pharmacist "to give bulk to minute doses of very active medicines administered in the form of a pill."

Nearly a century ago, *The Complete Herbalist* suggested the use of bread charcoal as a dentifrice: "Pulverize it (charcoaled bread) until it is reduced to an impalpable powder, then apply daily, morning and night, with a soft brush and pure cold water. This will keep the teeth white and cure diseases of the gums."

White bread is not a pure food; it is a poor food.

BUCKWHEAT

Along with such herbs as Rue, Elder, and Forsythia, this food has long been known to be a source of an invaluable principle, rutin, which in recent years has been of great service in medicine. Prof. Heber W. Youngken declares that rutin decreases capillary fragility and reduces recurrent hemorrhage that goes along with it.

True, Buckwheat is a good food only if it's 100% Buckwheat, not pearled, not refined and not as an insignificant part of a combination of Rye, Corn and other ground cereals. In its unrefined state and raised organically, it is an excellent source of Vitamin B and chlorine, iron, magnesium, phosphorus, potassium, sodium and sulfur. For best nutritional results, steam the food, do not overcook and do not include in soups or stews; and do combine it with non-starchy vegetables, not with starches or proteins.

"*Rutin:* A substance that occurs in Vitamin C in foods. It

is used in concentrated form for a treatment for high blood pressure. We suggest you get it from fresh raw fruits and vegetables." *Prevention.*

BUTTER

Use unsalted butter as a jiffy remedy for all kinds of recent burns. See under Ointment Bases and Lard. Since butter is a rich source of cholesterol, eat very little or none, the better to prevent the deposits of this substance from hardening the blood vessels. (See under Olive Oil).

Butter Used as Ointment

Today we are so accustomed to having butter around and to using it as a food, that the ancient history of butter will come as a shock. The Hindus offered butter as a sacrifice in their worship. The Greeks and Romans had butter but they didn't eat it. They used it as a remedy for injuries to the skin. They believed too, that the soot of burned butter was good for sore eyes. The Romans also used butter as an ointment for the skin and hair. In Spain, as late as the 17th Century, butter was found in medicine shops only! While the Hindus did use butter as a food about 2,000 years before Christ, very few people in early times regarded it as a food. And when it was eaten, it was generally used to enrich cooked foods. *News Report.*

"God has placed the most nourishing of the minerals in the skins of the fruit and vegetables we discard." . . . "The longer a man lives, the more he realizes how much his early ignorance has shortened his life. But unfortunately, when he wakes up, it is often too late to correct his mistakes."

Frederick W. Collins.

CABBAGE

This is a most inexpensive and excellent protective food, rich in the required vitamins of A, B, C, and especially the anti-ulcer Vitamin U, and possessing a good percentage of calcium, iodine and potassium and a higher one of chlorine and sulfur. The latter two minerals help greatly to cleanse the mucous membrane of the stomach and intestines. However, all this is possible only if the vegetable is consumed in its *uncooked* state, or its *fresh* juice drunk. It must be noted that if the outer leaves are discarded, a greatly needed abundance of calcium will be lost; if the vegetable is cut, slawed or shredded, much of the Vitamin C content will be needlessly lost through oxidation by (exposure to) the air. It is interesting to note that our early seamen when travelling long voyages, ate much of fresh Broccoli, Cabbage and Cauliflower as their means of preventing scurvy. To preserve its edibleness, the pith of the cabbage was scooped out and the vegetable was suspended with string and each morning the pith was filled with fresh water.

As for its medicinal virtues, Cabbage was used by the Roman physicians as a near cure-all, for headache, colic, deafness, drunkenness, insomnia and internal ulcers. And in this country, the food was steeped as a remedy for scurvy because of its high Vitamin C content, lack of appetite and nervous disorders, for which calcium and sulfur are often prescribed by the medical doctors. As an application to an abscess, one writer believed that a leaf dipped into hot water and applied to the affected area will bring "remarkable results." An eminent English physician earlier in the century highly recommended the French Formula for Chest Ailment. This was simply a decoction of red Cabbage in water to which an equal amount of Honey was added to make the "pectoral syrup." (And the French generally referred to this remedy as the English Formula.)

Late in 1953, there appeared certain news reports to show the efficacy of freshly prepared Cabbage juice as an anti-ulcer factor. One reporter in examining the facts stated: "Some progressive medical doctors are beginning to see the light, that is, they are commencing to realize that Hippocrates was right when he said: 'Let food be your medicine.' The value of raw cabbage juice in the cure of ulcers is now recognized by many regular medical practitioners."

Cabbage-juice potion helpful in ulcer cases

Researchers at Stanford University School of Medicine have

developed a cabbage-juice concentrate that appears to speed the healing of peptic ulcers and to reduce painful symptoms quite soon after administration. Vitamin U, an unidentified factor that is supposed to protect the digestive tract from pepsin, is believed to cause the beneficial action of the concentrate.   *News Report.*

Ulcer Cure Aided by New Vitamin

Cabbage juice containing vitamin U speeds recovery of patients with peptic ulcers, according to Dr. Garnett Cheney of the department of medicine, Stanford University medical school, here. An earlier paper by Dr. Cheney had indicated success in treatment of animals. Dr. Cheney reports that the administration of fresh cabbage juice to seven patients with duodenal ulcers resulted in a recovery within an average of 10.3 days. In contrast, he says, 62 patients reported in the literature showed a recovery in 37 days with standard therapy. In six other patients with gastric ulcers, the crater healing time with cabbage juice was only 7.3 days, as compared with 42 days for six patients reported in the literature treated by standard therapy.

"The rapid healing time of peptic ulcers observed in patients treated with fresh cabbage juice indicated that the active peptic ulcer dietary factor may play an important role in the genesis of peptic ulcers in man." The results of Dr. Cheney's tests were positive, though wider experiments and further study are advisable. All patients showed rapid improvement; the average healing time for the total of thirteen cases was nine days. Dr. Cheney states, "The results in this small series of cases are sufficiently encouraging to warrant treating a large group of carefully controlled patients with the anti-ulcer factor. At present such a study must be purely on an experimental basis."

It was considered important to note that cabbage is not the sole source of the anti-ulcer factor; for the latter is present in varying concentration in a variety of fresh greens and cereal grasses as well as in certain vegetable fats.

"Noteworthy is the fact that the anti-peptic ulcer factor which is readily destroyed by heat indicates that the preparation of food for human consumption by heating or cooking may completely destroy this factor. And if such is the case it would appear necessary to include certain raw foods in the diet of peptic ulcer patients, not only to promote the healing of ulcers

but to prevent the development of lesions in the future." (My italics.)   *News Report.*

❦   ❦   ❦

Nutrition Notes reports that Cabbage, Spinach and other green leafy vegetables contain Vitamin K which helps blood to clot. A deficiency of Vitamin K, which may greatly prolong clotting time, is rare because the body ordinarily synthesizes the vitamin. Nevertheless there is evidence that man cannot entirely dispense with food containing Vitamin K.

❦   ❦   ❦

CAMPHOR

The Camphor to be used is the pure, and not the synthetically prepared item that is used by the druggist for his preparations and that is marked U.S.P. (The "Camphor Balls" once used as a moth deterrent, are now actually naphthalene, contain no camphor and must be used only for that spring-cleaning chore. And for that purpose, the pure Camphor will prove far more effective).

Camphor has been used in medicine as a circulatory stimulant and it is more noted for its calmative influence in certain types of hysteria, general nervousness and neuralgia. But I do not recommend such usage for the laymen. We should be more interested in its external applications, for it is widely employed as an anodyne and counter-irritant for rheumatic affections, muscular sprains, bronchitis and other inflammatory conditions. It is frequently used for its anaesthetic effects to relieve itching of the skin, for which purpose the following is a typical remedy: Dissolve a half teaspoonful of camphor in a little alcohol and mix into 4 ounces of plain Calamine Lotion. Shake the mixture well before using.

Camphor Liniment: Dissolve ½ ounce of Camphor in 2 ounces of Olive Oil previously warmed slightly. (Any cooking oil will do.) Use as an anodyne lotion or embrocation, or as a substitute for the druggist's Camphorated Oil. 2. Dissolve ½ ounce of Camphor in 2½ ounces of 90% alcohol and add ½ ounce of vinegar.

Camphor and Turpentine Liniment: Dissolve an ounce of

Camphor in 8 ounces of turpentine. This may be used alone or combined in equal parts with Liniment. 1. Use as a stimulating embrocation for aching muscles. 2. Warm the turpentine slightly and add a teaspoonful of cut Cayenne Peppers. Allow to macerate for 2 days and add the Camphor. Strain and use as above indicated.

Camphor Water: Pour a pint of boiling water (distilled or rain preferred) upon ½ ounce of Camphor previously cut into small pieces, cover and allow to cool. Keep in a well-stoppered bottle. When needed, filter the liquid through filter-paper.

Williams Eye Water: The druggist dissolves 16.5 grams of pure Borax, U.S.P., in 1000 c.c. of Camphor Water (or 8 grains to each ounce) to produce a quart of this old-timer. The kitchen chemist approximates the amount of Borax by measuring ⅛ of a level teaspoonful of this powder and dissolving it in an ounce of Camphor Water. Filter the finished product. (60 grains=1 teaspoonful).

Camphor Compress: This is used as a local application to the closed eyes when they are tired or strained and to the forehead, for mild and temporary headaches. Mix equal parts of Camphor Water and Witch Hazel and apply as a compress.

Dr. Brown's Chilblain Ointment: The ingredients are ½ cup lard, 2 tablespoonsful turpentine, and ¼ ounce of finely ground Camphor. Dissolve the Camphor in the turpentine and gradually incorporate the latter with the lard.

Vaporizing Cream: The aforementioned remedy, being a loose cream, may well serve as an opportune Vaporub-substitute to help hasten the loosening of chest congestion. It may therefore, be modified by gradually adding ½ ounce of Spirits of Peppermint and/or 5 or 6 drops of Oil of Eucalyptus, and perhaps be even more effective.

Camphor Cream: Prepare the above remedy with all ingredients except the turpentine, in either a base of chicken fat, goose grease, mutton suet or lard.

🌷　🌷　🌷

CARAWAY

Caraway seeds serve as a culinary ounce of prevention by aiding the proper digesting of starchy though nourishing foods, as Cabbage, Turnip and Potatoes, and in this way, become a decided factor in preventing the possible formation of catarrh along the alimentary canal. The seeds are generally sprinkled over the dough of rye, pumpernickel and Swedish bread. They are also included in recipes of stews and soups of the Hungarian Goulash, Russian borscht, and plain Cabbage soup varieties; and they serve admirably with baked or boiled Potatoes, Apple sauce, pickled Beets, and in Squash and Pumpkin pie. And what is Sauerkraut or steamed Cabbage without a sprinkle of Caraway Seeds?

The medicinal virtues are today identified as anti-colic and carminative, for which purpose they have been employed for centuries. Herbal authorities of the 1600's, Mr. Nicholas Culpepper and John Parkinson, had this to say as to Caraway's remedial benefits: Mr. Culpepper, "Caraway confects, once only dipped in syrup (i.e., sugar and water) and one teaspoonful of them eaten in the morning and fasting and as many after each meal, is a most admirable remedy for those that are troubled with stomach colic." And Mr. Parkinson, "The seed is much used . . . with comfits that are taken for the cold and wind in the body, as also served for the table with fruit."

In Dr. Meyrick's *Family Herbal*, we read that the Caraway seeds, bruised, are good in hysteria and fits. Today it is recognized that many a hysteria or nervous condition can be traced to functional (stomach) disorders, which in turn are corrected more by proper dietary habits than by severe medication. And in turn "proper dietary habits" ask that Caraway seeds act as preventative medicine by being ingested with the nourishing, starchy Cabbage, Potato, et al, and non-nourishing pastries.

Antacid: Caraway Seeds, Fennel Seeds, Peppermint, and Spearmint. Directions: Take a half teaspoonful of each and stir well in a cup of hot water. Cover 10 minutes. Stir and strain. Drink one such entire cupful 4 times a day.

This infusion, carefully strained, is well suited to counteract the colic and flatulence of infants or small children.

🌷   🌷   🌷

CARROT

The Carrot is a wonderfully all purpose protective food and should be eaten as an uncooked vegetable, not via cole slaw, to provide the needed nutrients. A glassful of Carrot juice should be considered a *complete meal*, must be sipped slowly and carefully swished around the mouth to insure complete digestion and assimilation. The saliva is actually the first stomach enzyme that all food must encounter, and is referred to as ptyalin.

However, the warning not to over-drink on Carrot juice must be heeded. The roots contain a considerable proportion of the reddish pigment carotin or carotene, which is found also in Tomatoes, Pumpkins and other foods. It is a great mistake to believe that the ingestion of 2 glasses of Carrot juice at one time will be twice as beneficial as one glass. Not only will indigestion and general distress occur, but it may lead to a condition known as Carotinemia, in which the skin assumes a distinctly yellowish hue simulating jaundice.

Dr. Withering, of Digitalis fame, stated that the seeds of the Carrot freshly collected and dried were "to be used as diuretics and to disperse wind in the stomach, and there are many instances of their affording relief in (removing) the stone and gravel" (from the kidney apparatus.) A medical contemporary believed that these seeds "operate powerfully by urine, and are excellent in obstructions of the viscera, the jaundice and in the beginning of dropsies. A poultice of the roots has been found to mitigate the pain of foul cancerous ulcers, and take away the intolerable stench, . . ."

Indeed many medical compendia written since Withering's 18th century days contain formulae involving the Carrot. And where there appears a remedy in the form of a poultice or ointment, let it remind us of the druggist's Ointment of Vita min A & D. (The carotene ingredient later becomes Vitamin A.) And well do I recall Grandfather Isaiah's use of thin slices of Carrot root as an external application to leg ulcers.

Infusion of Carrot Seeds: Infuse ½ ounce in a pint of hot water and cover until cold. Stir and strain. This is taken during the day as a diuretic in dropsy and nephritic complaints.
Dr. Griffith.

Cataplasm of Carrot Root: 1. Scrape the root of a garden Carrot down to a pulp. Use as a fresh application to sore and foul ulcers. 2. Boil long enough to soften a root and mash. Apply and use as an emollient poultice.

Carrot Ointment: The ingredients are ½ pound of cut Carrot Root, 10 ounces of unsalted Lard and 1 ounce of yellow wax. Heat them together until the water of vegetation is driven off and the fat has acquired a yellow color. Then strain for use.   *After Dr. W. Proctor.*

Extract of Carrot Root: Take an amount of the juice of the Carrot Root and evaporate it slowly on very slow heat to a consistency of Honey. Use this extract as an application to ulcerated areas.

Violinist Says Juice Gives Vim: Joseph Szigeti, violinist, keeps fit by eating carrots whenever he gets "that tired feeling" during the course of his concert tours. More often he uses a juicer on the carrots, seasoned with a little spinach or a few dandelion leaves. Szigeti sticks to this routine for increased energy during all his exhausting tours which keep him busy 10 months out of the year.

🌷   🌷   🌷

CASHEW

Cashew nuts should always be eaten *un-roasted* for then they are wholesome and nutritious, but when boiled in oil and salted, there's always the danger of increased indigestion. This alkaline food is best combined with acid fruits and non-starchy vegetables, *not* with sweet fruits, proteins and starchy items. "The Brazilians are the only people," says Dr. Esser, "who fully appreciate the Cashew. It is used as a food and a household remedy by the poor, as a refreshing beverage by the sick, and as a sweetmeat on the tables of the wealthy."

There have been many uses for the oil of Cashew Nut. An early edition of *The Dispensatory* states that it used to be considered as "a discutient (an agent which causes the dispersal of a tumor or any pathological accumulation). In the West Indies the juice (or the active oil) is said to be employed in the treatment of ringworm. The oil of cashew-nut hulls has been employed in the treatment of leprosy." Dr. Meyrick had also written in the mid 1700's: "The shell abounds with an acid oil which cures tetters, ringworm, and other like eruptions by only anointing them therewith."

🌷   🌷   🌷

CASTOR OIL

The laxative or cathartic effects of this oil are too well known for further comment, but one should learn to appreciate more fully its other uses especially indicated for external application. The herbalist recognizes its emollient effects in seborrhea and other skin diseases.

Since Castor Oil has the advantage over other oils of being soluble in alcohol, it may be used as a hair tonic. The following preparation is considered of great value to heal irritations of the scalp and as an "antiseptic hair tonic." In a pint of alcohol, steep for one week, ¾ ounces each of Sage and Nettle; then strain and slowly add 2½ ounces of the oil to the alcohol.

Castor Oil is frequently used by the laymen as a wart reducer and corn solvent for which purpose a drop is placed upon the wart or corn several times a day if convenient, and covered with a bandage or Bandaid. The oil is used more extensively by the pharmacist and chemist to prepare an ointment which soothes irritations of the skin or chafing of infants. For this purpose, the oil is mixed with enough of equal parts of powdered corn starch and zinc oxide to make a smooth paste. The oil may also be mixed only with zinc oxide ointment.

Herbal Hair Tonic: Rosemary, 1 ounce; Nettle, ½ ounce; Sage, 2 ounces; Olive Oil, 1 ounce; Castor Oil, 1 ounce; Alcohol Ethyl (50%), 1 pint. Directions: The finely ground herbs are allowed to stay mixed in the alcohol for about a week. Then strain the mixture and add the oils and only enough water until there is produced a very slight turbidity. (See also under Olive Oil.)

🌷   🌷   🌷

CATNIP

As we all know, Mr. Felix the Cat enjoys this herb as a delightful tonic which seems to exert a stimulating and almost inebriating effect on Felix. And the effect upon the human— disappointing as it may be to some—is neither stimulating nor inebriating. Catnip has proven its therapeutic worth for several hundreds of years as an antispasmodic, carminative and diaphoretic.

A warm infusion of Catnip and Fennel seeds (equal portions) will offer a reasonable facsimile of the drugstore elixir of Catnip and Fennel, which is well known as an anti-colic and carminative remedy. The dose for an adult or child is a half cupful of the warm infusion and for an infant, as much as it will drink from a 4 ounce bottle.

An eminent physician of George Washington's time, enumerating various benefits of friend Catnip, wrote that "it is good in nervous disorders and the young tops made into a conserve are serviceable in that troublesome complaint, the night-mare. It is a good female medicine and may be used with great advantage in hysteria and other fits." And other older medical authorities also attest that the herb catnip is efficacious in the treatment of infantile colic, the treatment of colds and febrile complaints and during painful menses. Chewing the leaves has been believed to relieve the pain of toothache.

Thus in feverish colds, to induce sweating, steep a teaspoonful each of Catnip, Boneset, Mint and Sage in a cupful of hot water for 10 minutes, keep the cup saucered. Stir and strain, and drink one such cupful every hour for 4 or 5 doses.

It has long been reported to be of great service in scarlet fever and measles, for which purposes a warm infusion of Catnip, Yarrow and Saffron (a teaspoonful each of the former two, ¼ of the latter, in a cupful of hot water) is drunk by the patient every hour.

Not only will equal portions of Catnip, Anise and Fennel seeds, prepared as a warm infusion, be of excellent service as a gentle carminative and antacid, the mixture deserves honorable mention as a worthy tea or coffee substitute for the bilious and dyspeptic.

For nervousness, insomnia and nervous headache, a mixture ½ tsp each of Valerian root, Skullcap and Catnip is steeped to prepare a warm infusion. This dose, a cupful, is drunk 3 times a day, one hour after meals and about ½ hour before retiring.

A toothache or gum boil remedy is easily prepared by mixing equal parts of ground Hops and Catnip flowers and ½ of that amount of Sassafras bark. Stir only enough hot water to thoroughly moisten one teaspoonful of the mixture and apply it, contained in suitable cloth, as a poultice to the affected area.

Tisane: Mix equal parts of Catnip, Linden flowers and leaves, Peppermint and Marjoram. Steep for 5 minutes one teaspoonful of this mixture in a cup of hot water. Stir, strain and sip. (See also under charcoal.)

🌺　　🌺　　🌺

CELERY

The therapeutic properties of the roots and seeds were well considered by the medical contemporaries of Dr. William Meyrick (as by many others these past 250 years) who recommended the roots as a quickly operating diuretic, being "good in fits of the stone or gravel, and in the viscera. A strong decoction of them is the most effectual preparation." The seeds present their therapeutics chiefly as a warm carminative, and so help to "dispense wind in the stomach and bowels." As a "cure" for rheumatism Dr. Joseph G. Richardson, M. D., in 1904 prescribed strong teas of Celery stocks and roots to be "drunk freely 3 or 4 times a day. *It should be used freely as an article of diet,* (and the) expressed juice (taken) for rheumatism or neuralgic pains." (My italics.)

In current medical compendia, one will find that "in ancient times," "in the Orient," "in the past century," the seeds of both Smallage and Garden Celery, whose properties include aromatic, diuretic, nervine and tonic were employed as a medicine principally for upset stomach and especially as a nerve sedative to insure restful sleep. It was true in those days; it is true today. In recent years such therapeutics have been well demonstrated by researchers of food and pharmaceutical laboratories to be due chiefly to two all-important ingredients: the oil of Celery containing apoilin and the various factors of the Vitamin B Complex group.

Nervous Headache or Sleeplessness: ¼ teaspoonful each of Celery seed and Valerian and ½ each of Catnip and Skullcap. Prepare a warm tisane of the herbs in a cup of hot water. Allow to stay covered 10 minutes, stir and strain. For nervousness or headache, sip slowly one such cupful 3 or 4 times a day, and to overcome sleeplessness, one hour before retiring.

The juice of the fresh vegetable contains the much needed organic sodium which helps to maintain calcium in solution at a 4-1 ratio and therefore the proper fluidity of the blood (and lymph) and to prevent it from becoming too thick. There is also present in the fresh juice a high percentage of magnesium and iron, which helps to strengthen the blood cells. Eat Celery uncooked, either alone or with other vegetables or simple protein, not with fruits.

Please: Do not discard the pale green leaves of your own garden-grown produce, nor abuse their employment as a Parsley-like garnish. They are a must ingredient of vegetable (uncooked) salads and may well replace the familiar stalks, than which they are more tasty and as nourishing. Also it is best not to shred this excellent food; neither the leaves or stalks are to be incorporated into a cole slaw, truly a culinary monstrosity, nor even cut it up into 2-3 inch segments since such reduction in size results in a like reduction of the content of the much needed Vitamins. Above all, DO NOT COOK celery—Eat it as is, leaf and stalk, and *chew well,* thus you will conserve its wonderful food values. Moreover, the unhealthy habit of adding the synthetic, chemical salt is to be discouraged and the earlier in life the better, for indeed a mouthful or two of this highly, organically mineralized food supplies an adequate daily ration of sodium and chlorine.

If yours is store bought, remember that this food generally has been sprayed with toxic chemicals and to avoid possible accumulation or even traces of such harmful poisons, it is advised to soak the entire stalks in a weak solution of sodium bicarbonate for a minute or two (½ teaspoon to a basin of water, about a quart) and rinsing twice again in fresh, cold water.

In the Fall Celery plants may be "borrowed" from the garden and stored in the cellar, near a *clean* window which faces the morning to mid-day sun. Properly rooted in moist, rich garden soil, they will continue all winter to produce tender shoots for food and flavor.   From *Better Health with Culinary Herbs.*

CHARCOAL

For best results, this item when bought must be labeled:

Wood Charcoal or Activated Charcoal *U.S.P.* It is easily prepared by charring soft woods like Willow or Bass (Linden), powdering the prepared charcoal, and sifting the powder. Such wood burning must be done out of doors.

There have been many uses for Charcoal, a few of which *The Dispensatory* listed in early editions:

In diseases of the stomach it may be employed with advantage not only to absorb fermentative gases but also to overcome hyperacidity. In the intestinal tract it will remove many irritating substances, such as the toxic amines and organic acids of decomposed foods, probably also bacteria themselves. Dietzel has also shown that absorption of bacteria on the particles of charcoal, with a consequent germicidal effect, can take place. Numerous surgeons have reported on its value as a dressing for suppurating wounds of various types. Nahmmacher highly recommends the intrauterine application of charcoal in various forms of endometritis, especially in infected abortions. Charcoal poultices have long been used to absorb the odors from gangrenous and other foul wounds.

Among the many important medicinal uses for charcoal special attention may be called to its value as an antidote in various forms of poisoning, especially mercuric oxide, strychnine, phenol, (carbolic acid), mushroom and poisons for which we have not an efficient neutralizer.

Leschke says, according to *The Dispensatory*, that absorption therapy using carbon medicinals (wood charcoal) is the best treatment for mercury bichloride poison and most other oral poisons.

Dyspepsia Remedy: 1. Prepare an infusion of Catnip or Mint, to which is added a teaspoonful of powdered charcoal and mix well. Take one such dose every hour as required for dyspepsia, hyperacidity and nausea. 2. Stuff the powder into empty #00 gelatin capsules, which are obtainable at drug stores. Take one or two with warm Catnip or Mint tea as above described.

Cataplasm of Charcoal: 1. Mix a heaping teaspoonful of the powder into a cupful of Chamomile and prepare a poultice with warm water. This remedy is indicated as an application to foul and gangrenous ulcers. 2. Mix a teaspoonful with a cup of Oatmeal and apply as a poultice to ulcerated areas.

Charcoal Liquid: To ½ ounce of powder, slowly incorporate 2 ounces of glycerine and to this mixture add 8 drops of Spirits of Peppermint and enough water to make 8 ounces. Take a teaspoonful as needed.

Charcoal Tablets Improve 76 Patients with Acne

"Therapy with charcoal tablets—in addition to local and purenteral medication—constitutes a special and beneficial approach to the treatment of patients with acne *vulgaris,*" declares Dr. Rudolph S. Lackenbacher, of Chicago.

In a study of 100 patients with the disease, Dr. Lackenbacher administered Charcoal Tablets 3 times a day after meals. This was the only form of oral medication used, and dosage was often reduced to 2 tablets daily after 2 weeks, depending on the patient's response, he says. As a result of this treatment, 76% of the patients showed great improvement, Dr. Lackenbacher states, and moderate improvement was obtained in 24%. No side effects were observed, he adds, and all of the patients obtained some "amelioration in the size and number of acne efflorescences under this kind of therapy (with charcoal tablets)."

News Report.

❦　　❦　　❦

CHERRY

Cherry juice, or the liquid expressed from the fresh ripe fruits, has long served in medicine as a cold remedy; its high percentage (10) of malic acid yields a fever-reducing remedy, when administered with warm water, or in an herbal tea of Boneset or Catnip. Equal parts of the expressed juice and Honey provide one with a worthwhile cough remedy, a teaspoonful of this mixture being sipped every hour as needed.

These alkaline fruits are rich in Vitamins A, B, and C, Citric, lactic and succinic acids, and abound in minerals of calcium, magnesium, phosphorus, potassium, silicon, and sulfur. According to a noteworthy commentator of former years, the gum which is found on the trunk and branches of the Cherry Tree, served most admirably as a food substitute. "The garrison," wrote this authority, "consisting of more than a hundred men were kept alive during a siege of 2 months, without any other food than this gum, a little of which they frequently took in their mouths, and let it to dissolve gradually." The gum was also employed as mild remedy for kidney disorders, "strangury, heat of urine," etc.

A book of medicine written some 200 years ago states that the kernels were supposed to possess "very great and singular efficacy in apoplexies, palsies and nervous disorders in general; and a water distilled from them was long made use of as a remedy for these fits which young children are frequently troubled with."

Dr. Otto Raubenheimer, herbalist extraordinaire, informed me several years ago that he considered the stems of the Cherry fruits as a valuable remedy for asthmatic or bronchial conditions. A small handful, recommended the Doctor, were to be steeped in a pint of hot water until cold, strained and prepared into syrup with sugar or Honey. The prescribed dose was a tablespoonful every hour as needed.

Dr. Ludwig W. Blau, M. D., in the 1950 *Texas Reports on Biology and Medicine*, considered the eating of Cherries an effective means of treating gout and arthritis. Both canned Cherries, black or Royal Anne, or fresh Black Bing varieties (and also Cherry juice) were employed in the treatment with such favorable results that not only did the uric acid of the blood drop to its normal average but in the 12 cases where patients had a non-restricted diet but ate a half a pound of canned or fresh cherries each day none suffered an attack of gouty arthritis.

In *Food Field Reporter,* Nov. 10, 1958, there appeared a similar article, saying that "new evidence that canned cherry juice may relieve gout, gouty arthritis and similar ailments. . . . Dentists have been suggesting cherry juice to their patients and one of them found it useful in the treatment of pyorrhea."

Please: Eat only fresh Cherries. The canned fruits are generally heavily laden with white sugar and preservatives which makes it an unwholesome article of food.

❧   ❧   ❧

CHICKEN FAT

See under Ointment Bases and Lard.

CHIVES

Like cousins Onion and Garlic, Chives were employed in the more backward European countries to protect one against the Evil Eye and all diseases in general. In fact, besides being used by Romany Gypsies in their fortune-forecasts, all cousins were considered to be "magnets of the plague." That is, not only would a sufferer of consumption or influenza drink hot infusions of Onions or Chives, he deemed it imperative that a clump of Chives be suspended from the center of the sick room and from as well—in most cases—a bed-post within reach. This practice, so guaranteed the fortune-tellers, was a sure means of drawing to the Chives "maladies that would otherwise fall on the inmates."

Years ago, Chives were employed, either alone or in combination with the more pungent Onion and Garlic, as a medicinal remedy for the "nervous" bronchial disorders and especially for blood diseases. The discreet inclusion of uncooked Chives in one's meals guarantees a most complete assimilation of the greater percentage of this plant's health sustaining nutrients: An excellent source of Vitamin C and to a lesser degree, vitamins A, B, and G. Minerals are the blood fortifiers sulfur and iron. It is this sulfur's component which is somewhat similar to cousin Garlic's, being the active bactericidal crotonaldehyde, a worthy defender of the nasal and respiratory areas against disease. (Is that why Garlic-eating Italians rarely are asthma victims?) Moreover, the members of the Chive family stimulate the saliva and digestive juices while at the same time performing the duties of intestinal antiseptics. A syrup of Chives (or better of Onion or Garlic) serves well as a cold cough remedy especially useful in croup or spasms of asthma.

🌷   🌷   🌷

"Rest a little as you go along life's path. This may save a total collapse in your sunset days."

🌷   🌷   🌷

"The average person eats too much and chews too little."
                                                        Mark Twain.

🌷   🌷   🌷

CINNAMON

Since ancient Biblical days has Cinnamon been used as a preservative, medicine and flavoring seasoning spice. It was a principal ingredient of the anointing oil and disinfectant mixtures used in the Holy Temples of the Hebrews.

Today, it is employed in medicine and pharmacy as an efficient aromatic, being warm and cordial to the stomach and intestines. Its therapeutic effects are described as being carminative, anti-nausea, and relieving of painful flatulence. It has also been recommended in diarrhea, due to its distinctly astringent nature.

However, it should be used with care and moderation, and only in the absence of other remedial agents. To be sure this much used spice has merit, but an overdose will create the same internal hazard which is so often incurred by Cloves and Ginger and other spices.

For the chronic dyspeptic, Cinnamon water will prove an effective remedy if taken tepid-warm and in tablespoonful doses. It is prepared by stirring a quarter teaspoonful of the ground spice in a cupful of hot water. Cover with a saucer for 15 minutes and again stir. Strain carefully. For variation, a few Caraway or Cardamon seeds or culinary herb as Catnip or Marjoram may be added to the steeping liquid.

Compound Cinnamon Water: Mix equal parts of ground Cinnamon, Fennel seeds, ground Catnip and Sage. Stir well a teaspoonful in a cup of hot water and cover for 10 minutes. Stir and strain. Dose: One-two tablespoonsful as required to relieve stomach colic and spasm, flatulence, etc.

Gargle: Take one tablespoonful of each: Ground Sage and Cinnamon, and Sumac berries. Boil the Sumac berries in a pint of hot water for a half hour, add the Sage and Cinnamon and simmer another ¼ hour. Stir and strain. Gargle warm every ½ hour or as often as required.

A jiffy deodorizer that will quickly dispel undesirable odors is easily prepared by boiling a few pieces of Cinnamon in a quart of hot water. Grandfather used to sprinkle a little of the powder on the hot stove.

Tea Substitute: Actually, the above remedies, Cinnamon water and Compound Cinnamon water are examples of herb teas, or Tisanes, as the herbalist calls them. The other herbs that have been previously recommended as co-partners with Cinnamon are Cardamon, Fennel, Catnip, Sage and Marjoram. Those who are susceptible to the dyspepsiating tannic acid and the over-stimulation of the caffeine of tea and coffee will do well to remember that an herb tea is a "health tea." The writer has known one particular confirmed coffee drinker (c.c.d.) who gradually forsook this negative dietary habit by this simple procedure: At first, the c.c.d. placed a 4-5 inch long stick of Cinnamon in his cup of hot coffee frequently stirring the stick of spice in the coffee which he sipped with measured anticipation (and some bewilderment). Upon the herbalist's recommendation, he undertook the drinking of tisanes of Sage, Mint, etc., used Cinnamon less and less frequently and in time, was a practitioner of the true faith and herb-tea drinking and no longer an addict of the twin stimulants, tea and coffee. Credit must be given the c.c.d.'s will power and determination to seek better health by living within and conforming to the laws of Natural Hygiene, Natural foods, better eating habits, no salt, vinegar or spices with foods, fresh air and exercise and especially more sleep and restful habits.

Compound Wine of Cinnamon: Simmer for 10 minutes ¼ teaspoonful each of Cinnamon, Clove, Mace and Cardamon in a pint of warmed wine. Allow to cool, strain and add 10 ounces of sugar.

Use as a cordial stomachic and anti-colic in flatulence, in teaspoonful doses mixed in a little warm water. (See under Milk).

❦   ❦   ❦

CLOVES

Medicinally Clove oil has been much employed in medicine as an anesthetic in toothache, as a stimulating expectorant in bronchial disorders, and as a powerful germicide and antiseptic. The housewife, too, has profited by its persistent pungency which has proven to be such an invaluable aid in pickling Watermelon rinds. But Cloves as a seasoning agent should not be used to flavorize your foods.

The whole, unground Cloves, (technically the flower buds) have long been recommended and used as a stimulating carminative for the relief of severe flatulence and indigestion.

For this purpose, 2 or 3 Clove buds are allowed to steep in a cup of hot water for several minutes, and the resulting solution, strained, is sipped slowly while moderately warm or tepid. Cloves are a must with an herbalist friend who insists that the buds be steeped together with pekoe tea.

Clove Water: Add 2 teaspoonsful of Cloves to a pint of hot water, allow to macerate for ½ hour in a covered vessel and strain. Take a tablespoonful (warm or with warm water) as often as needed as a stimulating carminative in flatulence.

Prepared as a decoction, this solution possessing the characteristic strong, fragrant odor of the spice has proven to be a most effective deodorizer for a sick room. The vessel containing the warm liquid should be placed upon the warm radiator. And a few Cloves may also be used in a vaporizer, as a substitute for Tincture of Benzoin Compound or other vaporizing solution.

We have used Cloves as an effective moth preventive and Camphor substitute by combining them with Lavender, Wormwood and Tansy, and as an ingredient of sachets and potpourris.

🌼　　🌼　　🌼

Good Diet Halts Tooth Decay

Evidence is growing that mineral elements other than fluorides can make substantial contributions to protetction against tooth decay, according to Dr. C. G. King, executive director of the Nutrition Foundation. Initial evidence indicates, he says, that sufficient sources of those extra mineral intakes are furnished in a normal supply of such foods as meats, leafy vegetables, and whole grains. Hence, Dr. King notes, "There is sound reason to emphasize the importance of over-all diet as being a protective factor against tooth decay."　　　　*News Report.*

🌼　　🌼　　🌼

COCONUT

"In tropical countries," writes Dr. Esser, "where the Coconut Palm is grown, nearly every part of the tree is utilized by the natives. The roots are used as an astringent medicine, and are sometimes chewed as a substitute for betel or areca nuts, sometimes interwoven with fibers to form baskets. The trunk which, when mature, develops a very hard outer shell, is used to form rafters and pillars of native buildings. . . . The fully grown leaves are put to numerous uses: They are formed into mats, baskets, roof coverings for native huts, fences, articles of clothing and ornaments."

Eat this protein food with such acid fruits as Orange or Pineapple and vegetables, fresh and uncooked, and never with starch foods or other proteins.

The fresh meat of the Coconut is today considered by the medical laity as a "powerful taenicide (destroyer of tapeworm, acquired by eating insufficiently cooked meats of infested animals). The patient should drink the milk then eat the flesh of the nut." It is used especially in India as a general vermifuge.

❦   ❦   ❦

COD LIVER OIL

Ever since Cod Liver Oil gained recognition as a source of nutrient, it has entered into a variety of medicinal preparations and patent remedies. It has been used as an "alterative" in chronic rheumatism, under-nourishment, tuberculosis, respiratory diseases and in skin disorders.

The United States Dispensatory states that in past years, "Cod Liver Oil has attracted some attention as a local remedy for the treatment of burns and ulcers. Lint soaked with the oil is placed over the burned area and left in place for 48 hours, fresh oil being poured onto the lint as may be required, usually every 12 to 24 hours."

Ointment of Cod Liver Oil is of special benefit for surface wounds, poison ivy, burns, chafing and similar skin irritations of infants as well as adults, etc. One of the following preparations may be used: 1. Of Cod Liver Oil, Petroleum jelly (vaseline) and Lanolin, use equal parts and mix well to form a uniform ointment. 2. Mix equal portions of this with Zinc Oxide Ointment. If available, it is suggested to incorporate also, 25% Lanolin and 5% Beeswax, of the total quantity. 3. The ingredients are 3 ounces of Cod Liver Oil, 6 tablespoonsful of Spermaceti and 2 teaspoonsful of Beeswax. If latter two are unavailable, use an ounce of simple Cerate obtainable at your drugstore. Melt together and stir until cold. (See also under Lanolin).

COFFEE

In the early 1700's, coffee was in vogue principally as an "excellent remedy for those who are troubled with habitual headaches, arising from weakness of the stomach or contracted by hard drinking". And with the prescribing of this remedy, came the accompanying warning: "In delicate constitutions, it is apt to produce nervous symptoms." How true that is today!

Mr. Fish, formerly of the Worcester Electric Company, has stated that alternating doses of warm, diluted coffee and Pumpkin seeds were much employed in his family as a pin worm expellant. (Ed: No coffee for children, please.)

However, in cases of accidental poisoning due to barbiturates or bromides, the generally accepted antidote is coffee, two cupsful every 30 to 40 minutes, until stimulation is effected. In cases of narcotic poisoning, brewed coffee is also administered by rectal injection, the freshly brewed coffee being diluted with an equal portion of water.

As a medicine, the much more powerful caffeine, which is the active ingredient of coffee, has almost entirely replaced the use of the coffee bean.

COLD CREAM

See under Lard and Ointment Bases.

CORIANDER

Coriander was well known as a medicinal remedy to the Ancients and was listed in the Ebers papyrus. It was also mentioned in the writings of Cato and Pliny, by early Sanskrit writers, and in the Mosaic books, Exodus and Numbers. Its fruit, states the *Lloyd Bulletin*, was used by the Hebrews and the Romans as a medicine, as well as a spice, in very early days.

The seeds are much used today in seasoning foods. *The Dispensatory* declares that this "gentle aromatic offers its therapeutic services when combined with other medicines, either to cover their taste, to render them acceptable to the stomach, or to correct their griping qualities." Moreover, it is the carminative-plus ingredient of the excellent general tonic and stomachic, Compound Infusion Gentian, which according to the druggist's *National Formulatory*, contains Gentian root, Coriander and Orange peel. A somewhat similar home-made infusion is easily prepared by simmering a teaspoonful each of Gentian, Coriander and dried Orange or Lemon peels in a pint of boiling water for 10 minutes and straining the mixture when cool; and the dose, mixed in a wineglass of water, is sipped slowly 3-4 times a day. Coriander enters other "official" formulae of Tincture of Rhubarb Compound and the commercialized Confection of Senna. The latter preparation contains Senna, Coriander, Figs, Tamarinds, Prunes and Licorice and has been regarded as an effective and thorough laxative.

Coriander Water: Steep ⅔ teaspoonful in a cup of hot water 10 minutes, steam and drink the cupful whenever a carminative is needed.

❦   ❦   ❦

CORN SILK

When Corn is to be prepared for table use, it should be young, cooked in the jacket for 2 or 3 minutes and in very little boiling water and *thoroughly masticated* to insure the complete digestion of this starchy food. When picnicking this summer, be sure to roast a few young and tender ears in an open fireplace. [Yes, Irwin, a very small amount of butter (unsalted) may be added.] The older the Corn, the greater the depreciation in values of Vitamins C, A and B1, in that order. Thus, it is best to buy this food as fresh as possible, even if it means asking your farmer friends to remove the ears from the stalks, while you wait. The quick cooking of Corn and its complete mastication offer double assurance that these minerals will be available for assimilation: calcium and phosphorus, sodium and chlorine, magnesium and phosphorus.

"The new wonder drug, Nitrofurazone, better known as furacin, is made from corn cobs and is a powerful antibiotic. It has been used successfully as a germ killer in the treatment of various skin infections and wounds, to destroy disease-causing fungus and as an antihistamine in the treatment of the common cold and certain allergies." (See under Wheat.)

From the Fresh Corn, salvage the yellow silk, dry it well and store in a tin can. It has been used by the laity and pharmacists as a diuretic in cystitis, and in all disorders of the kidneys and bladder. (See under Asparagus.) For this purpose a teaspoonful of the finely cut silk is steeped in a cup of hot water, covered until cool and strained. One such cupful is drunk 4 times a day.

❧   ❧   ❧

CORN STARCH

It has been previously stated that a paste of powdered Starch and Castor Oil will be found useful to allay irritations of the skin, and here again, as in the case of the Oil, is another example of a common household item that possesses other medicinal properties.

To absorb excessive or irritant secretions, the powder may be dusted upon the skin, and for even better results, should be mixed with plain talc, in equal parts, thus preventing its forming an undesirable pasty mass with the absorbed fluid. What better baby powder is there than plain Corn Starch? Yes, Corn Starch is an ingredient of *Mexsana Powder* usually found in drugstores.

The following formula is used as a base of several medicinal pastes and is frequently prescribed by the physician for various skin disorders: 3 ounces each of Corn Starch and Zinc Oxide powder, 2 ounces of Glycerin and enough Lime Water to make a pint. Remember to shake the mixture well before using. When there is a condition of excessive itching, 2 teaspoonful of precipitated sulfur may be added to a pint of this lotion.

An enema of starch may be used as a demulcent injection in irritations of the rectum and may be prepared by mixing a tablespoonful of powdered starch in enough water to form a paste, then gradually adding more water to measure a pint. The enema may also be prepared by "dissolving" the powder in hot water, and allowing to cool. The mixture is boiled a few minutes and when cool, it is injected into the rectum. The starch preparation frequently offers quick relief of pain and discomfort caused by hemorrhoids and similar rectal disorders. The starch liquid has also served well as an antidote in Iodine poisoning.

Lassar's paste is composed of Corn Starch, Zinc Oxide and Petrolatum and is generally sold by druggists. It is used in various dermatologic conditions, as with Zinc Ointment, about which numerous medical authorities state that it has the advantage of adhering to the skin more satisfactorily. This preparation contains in 100 Grams (Gm.): Zinc Oxide powder 25 Gm. (approximately 1 ounce), Corn Starch 25 Gm., and White Petrolatum (Vaseline) 50 Gm. First mix the powders with a little mineral oil before they are added to the petrolatum.

❧   ❧   ❧

All "enriched" foods are as enriched as you are when a thief takes the cash out of your wallet and replaces it with a counterfeit substitute.

❧   ❧   ❧

CRANBERRY

The famous clipper ships out of Gloucester and New Bedford, sailing the Seven Seas for spices, teas and whale oil, invariably carried open wooden casks filled with tiny crimson berries. Nobody had heard of Vitamins and "ascorbic acid" in those days, but the captains of those sturdy little barks knew that the men under them kept healthier if plenty of fresh Cranberries, the fruit that grew so thickly in the bogs on Cape Cod, were included in the ship's stores. The sailors ate the raw berries—and stayed well, despite the lack of other fresh produce. Cranberries, thus, were the Yankee answer to scurvy, playing the same role as Lemons, (then called "limes") for English seamen.

The New England women also knew the value of using Cranberries. They made Cranberry sauce, of course, but they also used them in other ways. They made jams and jellies of the rich red fruit. They made spicy conserves and ketchups.   *Here's Health.*

Dr. Finkel tells us that the fruits are employed to "help contract a dilated stomach and are good for dysentery, flatulence and diarrhea. Also splendid for the removing of (blood) toxins and very effective in liver troubles, scurvy, and erysipelas. Cranberry drinks check fevers and asthma spasms."

Because of their tart taste, the fruits are generally not eaten fresh or in the uncooked state, but when overcooked or sugared, they become quite over-acid and then should be considered an undesirable food. But any excess of the fresh fruits may be frozen quickly and successfully: Pick over such fruits, discarding those that are soft or imperfect, wash and drain them. Place them in moisture resistant containers, seal and store in the freezer. To avoid indigestion or stomach distress, Cranberries must not be eaten with sugar, sweets or starches.

The medicinal claims attributed to these fruits have run into the dozens. Suffice it to say that only the following are acceptable: Poor complexion, pimples and skin diseases, bad blood and high blood pressure.

One informant tells me that in cases of boils and erysipelas, he had employed a poultice of crushed Cranberry fruits.

However, it has been the experience of the herbalist to gather and use the Summer collected leaves, dried and ground, as a substitute for Blueberry leaves (which see) as a diuretic for kidney ailments, and as an anti-diabetic remedy.

CRISCO

See under Lard and Ointment Bases.

CUCUMBER

The writers of other days had high praise for the medicinal virtues of Cucumbers. Said one, "It is of a cooling nature and good for such that have a hot bilious constitution, and wherever there is a tendency to inflammation. The seeds are accounted cooling and diuretic and beaten into an emulsion with barley water. They are good in the strangury and all other disorders of the urinary passages." And an herbal doctor of the 1600's strongly approved of the Cuke's being chopped, skin and all, and cooked with (unrefined) Oatmeal and eaten at breakfast, dinner and supper, this taken for 3 weeks without intermission. Such a diet, his experience over many years, "doth perfectly cure all manner of sauce flegme and copper faces, red and shining fieree noses with pimples, rubies and other such precious faces."

The freshly expressed juice was used by milady of high Roman society to "drown her sorrows." And several years ago there arose a fad of using the juice, either alone or combined with fresh Buttermilk, as a cosmetic to bleach the skin.

Dr. Pope tells us that the Cucumber is:

recognized as being probably the best natural diuretic known, secreting and promoting the flow of urine. It has other valuable properties, as the promotion of hair growth, due to its high silicon and sulfur content particularly when mixed with Carrot, Lettuce and Spinach juice. . . . The addition of Cucumber juice to Carrot juice has a very beneficial effect on rheumatic ailments resulting from excessive retention of uric acid in the system. . . . The high potassium content of Cucumber makes this juice very valuable in helping conditions of high and low blood pressure. It is equally helpful in afflictions of the teeth and gums, such as pyorrhea. Our nails and our hair need particularly the combination of elements which fresh vital Cucumber juice furnishes, helping to prevent the splitting of the nails and falling of the hair. Skin eruptions of many kinds have been helped by drinking Cucumber juice to which the juices of Carrot and Lettuce have been added.

The Cucumber becomes a good source of needed nutrients only if it is eaten uncooked or quickly steamed, unpeeled and unsalted. For your better digestion, eat very little or none of the vegetables that have gone through the pickling or salting process, for the resultant pickle, though flavored, offers food value next to nil.

In its natural state, the vegetable possesses the enzyme erepsin which like Papaya, helps to better digest proteins.

This vegetable has not only been a source of food nutritives and protein-digesting enzymes; indeed, it should be considered as an ingredient of a soothing ointment and cosmetic preparation. Cucumber jelly will also prove to be an excellent application for chapped hands, irritations and roughness of the skin.

Cucumber Hand Lotion, or Jelly

Irish Moss —one teaspoonful
Tragacanth —one teaspoonful
Borax —one teaspoonful
Boric Acid —one teaspoonful
Glycerin —2 ounces
Alcohol (70%)—3 ounces
Cucumber Juice 3 ounces
Water to make 16 ounces
Perfume as Desired.

Directions

The Tragacanth and Irish Moss are stirred well in a pint of hot water which when cool, is strained. In this liquid, dissolve the Borax and Boric Acid and add the Cucumber juice, glycerin and alcohol. Add enough water to make 16 ounces.

Note: The juice is extracted from the Cucumber by grinding it in a meat grinder.

Cucumber Ointment

Green Cucumber—one pound
(Fit for the table)
Unsalted Lard 3½ ounces
Suet —2 ounces

Directions

Add the expressed Cucumber juice slowly to the melted base and stir constantly. Keep adding to the ointment as it thickens, beating the juice in with a wooden spatula. Keep the ointment in a glass jar covered with Rose water prepared by decocting Rose petals, to prevent the access of air.

❧ ❧ ❧

CUMIN

The Cumin mentioned in the Bible (Isaiah 28:25 and 27

and Matthew 23:23) is the same Cumin of present day commerce that is used principally as a flavoring agent. The herb is also found in the writing of Hippocrates, Dioscorides and Pliny, as the seasoning agent in the homemade breads of their times and as a stimulating aromatizer of their sweetened mulled (spiced) wines.

In ancient days, it was of service as a carminative and anti-spasmodic but since there are far many more less expensive herbs, it is not in use today for remedial purposes. The following remedy has long been employed in the British Isles as a prevention of a disease of pigeons known as scabby breast. English herbalists and chemists (druggists) still recommend to pigeon fanciers, and for them prepare, a mixture of equal parts of Caraway, Cumin, Dill and Fennel seeds, of which a pinch or "just enough" is mixed in with flourmeal and baked to yield a food for the birds. In the last century, the Seeds were simmered with resins (the gummy exudations of trees) to make a warm stimulating plaster in veterinary surgery.

🌷   🌷   🌷

"If you want to know the man who keeps you from accomplishing things; if you want to know what holds you back; if you want to know where to fix the blame, get a looking-glass and look into it carefully."   *Dr. Carl Loeb.*

🌷   🌷   🌷

BLACK CURRANTS

It has been previously mentioned that Black Currant fruits, as well as dozens of other everyday fruits and vegetables, serve as medicinal remedies as well as much needed sources of health-fortifying nutrients.

Currants have been employed as a gargle and as an ingredient in a cough syrup and lozenges. To prepare a gargle for a throat irritation especially due to or associated with a cold, simmer but do not boil, for 10 minutes, two heaping teaspoonsful of the fruits in two full cups of hot water. Strain through absorbent cotton. Gargle ¼ of a cup of liquid content every hour, or oftener, if so desired. The solution may be rewarmed for the next dose.

A syrup is almost immediately obtained by dissolving a tablespoonful either of Honey or raw brown sugar in a cupful of the still warm gargle preparation. And as with other herbal cough remedies, the dose generally is: "Take as much as often as is required."

Many drugstores today sell the Allenbury's Glycerine and Black Currant pastilles which are made from the ripe fruits. The lozenges are intended to offer relief for "minor irritations of the throat and huskiness of the voice due to cold, exposure, wind and dust. These soothing and demulcent pastilles are entirely harmless and may be taken freely."

To prepare your own cough drops or lozenges, you may follow the general procedure for making molasses candy, or, if you have had the previous experience, for making Hoarhound drops. (See under Sugar.)

Dr. Meyrick tells us that the "juice of the berries boiled up with sugar affords a jelly (syrup) which is exceedingly useful in sore throats, particularly those of the inflammatory kind." This remedy may today be used for bronchitis. He also quotes a passage from Dr. Withering's writings, to wit: "The young roots infused in boiling water afford a useful liquor in fevers of the eruptive kind, which is also good for dysentery and flux in cattle."

To prepare an effective gargle, simmer 2 heaping teaspoonsful of the fresh fruits (or one of the dried) in a glassful of hot water for 10 minutes, add ½ teaspoonful of ground Cinnamon and cover ½ hour. Strain and use warm.

🌷   🌷   🌷

DATE

Arabs make full use of the date palm. The dates are eaten, and also fed to donkeys and camels; the date stones are ground into meal; date blossoms are made into a beverage; stale fruit is converted into a vinegar; leaves are woven into household articles, and stronger branches are used in making furniture. Date stones are used by children to play games.

Although the Date is a concentrated food, it is most

nourishing and easily digested. We often give our children a few dates instead of candy and recommend them to all parents, who must ever safeguard the health of children by giving them—or deceiving them with—a minimum of worthless, candy-store goodies. Dates are best eaten with sweet fruits, not with starches and protein. They contain high percentages of vitamins A, B, D, and G, (the B vitamins supply thiamin and riboflavin) and minerals of iron, calcium, chlorine, copper, magnesium, phosphorus, potassium, sodium and sulfur.

Medicinally, they have been used as a laxative. For this purpose they are either boiled in water, 6 to a pint of hot water, and the resultant liquid drunk warm, morning and night; or 5 or 6 may be eaten and then a glass of warm water drunk, this done also twice a day.

It should be consumed regularly each day as a remedial measure for these ailments: Poor circulation, piles, constipation, nervousness. (The material above is adapted from my radio broadcasts, *Foods Are Your Medicines.*)

The date is superior as a source of food salts, supplying seven times as much lime as does beef tenderloin. The date requires nothing but the simple addition of milk to constitute a complete diet. A pound of dates and a quart of (unpasteurized) milk afford nourishment not only sufficient in quantity to supply the needs of the average person for a day, but of the very highest quality.

American people are suffering greatly from lime (calcium) starvation, which is resulting not only in loss of stature, due to lack of bone development, but also in an almost universal premature decay of teeth. The free use of dates with milk as a part of the American breakfast would conduce greatly to the improvement of the national health and the lowering of the mortality rate."

> *John Harvey Kellogg,*
> founder of the Battle Creek Sanatoriums.

❉   ❉   ❉

Health and good estate of body are above all gold, and a strong body above infinite wealth.   *Bible.*

❉   ❉   ❉

DILL

In Biblical days, the herb Dill was highly prized as a seasoner of foods and as a medicinal remedy, and the Anise referred to in Matthew 23:23, is actually Dill. The Anethum found in the original Greek passage was incorrectly translated as Anise and has so appeared for the past 600 years.

The taste of Dill resembles Fennel but is slightly more pungent, and is an indispensable must for pickled Cucumbers and Beets. John Parkinson said, 1640: "It is also put among pickled cucumber where it doth very well agree, giving to the cold fruit a pretty spicie taste or relish." The seeds enter the preparation of green Apple pies and salmon hors d'oeuvres. Try them with soups and Beans, Cabbage, Cauliflower and Peas. If you are to use the seeds in cheese, as spreads or sandwich, let them stay stirred in the cheese (cottage or creamed) a day or two before serving.

Mr. Nicholas Culpepper, herbal authority of the 1600's had written: "The seed is of more use than the leaves, and more effective to digest raw and viscous humors, and is in medicines that serve to expel wind and pains proceeding therefrom." Today, several hundred years after Mr. Culpepper's time, Dill seeds (fruits) are used for the same medicinal purposes, only now the terms used are more impressive: Aromatic and Carminative, etc. Dill water was a favorite "grandmother's" remedy for nausea and stomach distress. However, for colic and flatulence of infants and the elderly, a mixture of equal amounts of Dill, Anise and Fennel in warm infusion is recommended (half teaspoonful to a cup of hot water). Hence, the derivation of the name Dill, which is said to have been derived from an old word, *dilla*, to lull, alluding to the soothing carminative properties of the plant. For this reason, Dill seeds should be combined with other stomachic preparations, especially laxatives.

Colic Remedy for Infants, Dill Water: This is easily prepared and will be found most satisfactory in preventing and quickly relieving the discomforts of colic. Steep ½ teaspoonful in a cup of hot water and cover for 5-6 minutes. Stir well and strain into a 4 ounce nursing bottle. Give about two ounces (or all 4 if the baby accepts the invitation) via either nipple or spoon.

For older children: Increase the amount of seeds according to age and prepare as before.

Carminative (Flatulence) Remedy: Prepare a tea of ¼ teaspoonful (more or less) each of Anise, Dill, Fennel and Catnip in a cup of hot water. Dose: A warm cupful sipped slowly 4 times a day . . . eating very little during the day.

❧   ❧   ❧

EGG

Please save your eggshells, for if you are a gardener or even an indoor horticulturist, eggshells, thoroughly dried and finely ground, are an admirable food source for your flowers and plants. They are indeed very much needed to fertilize Rose bushes and should be buried deep enough below the soil's surface, to keep them from being dug up by cats or dogs. Eggshells contain certain minerals intended to keep garden produce and other vegetation in a healthy condition.

Many coffee drinkers prepare this drink by crumbling the eggshell in the decoction while it is boiling, and others use the skin of the eggs for drawing boils, according to Mrs. Fannie Smith.

"An old-fashioned remedy for minor cuts or bruises: Apply the moist surface of the inside coating or skin of the shell of a raw egg. It will adhere of itself, leave no scar, and heal without pain."   *Let's Live.*

The egg has also been engaged as a simple home shampoo and hair conditioner for a child's hair. The hair, if very soiled, may be first washed quickly with soap, rinsed well, and then a well-beaten egg worked thoroughly into the scalp and hair. Allow it to remain a few minutes and rinse well, at least twice, with cool water. Some even use two egg applications instead of one of soap and one of egg.

Liniment of Egg: 1. Mix well one egg yolk with 2 ounces of Flaxseed oil; or 2. One egg white with 3 ounces of the oil. Use as an application for recent burns.

"Health is one's best asset in life. Disease (sickness) is always a liability."   *Dr. Harry Finkel.*

❧   ❧   ❧

FENNEL

A few notes on the historical background of herb Fennel reveal that its fruits and edible succulent shoots were utilized by the ancient Romans and Greeks and by the people before them. This herb was highly recommended by the great Greek physician, Hippocrates, and considered by Pliny to possess at least two-score remedies, some of which are herein discussed. Poet Longfellow alludes to one such virtue —of strengthening and restoring the eyesight:

> "Above the lower plants it towers,
> The Fennel with its yellow flowers;
> And in an earlier age than ours
> Was gifted with the wondrous powers,
> Lost vision to restore."
>
> From *Goblet of Life.*

"For to make one slender," *The Good Housewife's Jewell* (1585) recommended that one "take Fennel and seeth it in water, a very good quantity, and wring out the juice thereof when it is sod, and drink it first and last, and it shall swaze either him or her."

The insistence of Fennel's slenderizing agency was, in later years, to be corroborated by Herbalist William Coles (1650). He had stated in *Nature's Paradise:* "Both the seeds, leaves and root of our Garden Fennel are much used in drinks and broths for those that are grown fat, to abate their unyieldiness and cause them to grow more gaunt, and lank." Furthermore, it is quite probable that the Ancient Greeks knew well of the properties of this herb, for they called it *Marathon,* derived from *maraino,* to grow thin.

Fennel has generally been considered a must whenever fish is in order, especially salmon and mackerel, so that the rather indigestible, fatty oil of that food may be properly counter-balanced by the carminative, aromatic properties of the herb. Or as Mr. Culpepper aptly put it, "One good old custom is not yet left off, viz, to boil fennel with fish, for it consumes the phlegmatic humors which fish most plentifully afford and annoy the body with, *though few that use it know wherefore they do it.*" (My italics)

As for medicinal properties of Fennel, allow the conservative *United States Dispensatory* (XXII Ed.) [b]to admit that "Fennel seed is one of our most grateful aromatics . . . corrigent of other less pleasant medicines, particularly Senna and Rhubarb. In infants, the infusion was formerly employed as an enema of the expulsion of flatus. . . . Fennel water is a pleasant vehicle with a flavor suggestion of anise water." Prof. Youngken states that Fennel seeds (fruits) are to be used as a "stimulant, carminative, condiment and galactagogue." A carminative or anti-colic remedy is mentioned under Dill, which see.

For the useful new-fashioned proprietary Elixir of Catnip and Fennel, there may be substituted either the aforementioned or the following recipe: One teaspoonful composed of equal parts (or ¼ teaspoonful each of) Catnip, Chamomile, and Fennel or Mint, to be prepared and taken as a warm infusion 4-5 times a day as needed. This is suitable for infants and adults.

Fennel's virtue of "restoring" lost vision has been above described by Longfellow, since for centuries it had been recognized as an ingredient of eye lotions.

Eye Wash: Steep ⅛ teaspoonful each of Fennel, Chamomile and/or Eyebright, in a cupful of hot boiled water and cover until it is cold. Stir, strain and filter carefully through absorbent cotton. Wash eye with eye cup every 2-3 hours or as required.

Reducing Aid: Simmer for 5 minutes in 2 pints of boiling water ½ teaspoonful each of Licorice and Sweet Flag Roots, Kelp, Sassafras Bark and one of Fennel seed and Chickweed. Cover 15 minutes and strain. Take about ⅔ cupful (warm) morning, afternoon and evening.

Powdered Fennel occurs in the druggist's mildly laxative mixture, Compound Powder of Senna (formerly called Compound Powder of Licorice). In this formula, the herb acts as a soothing carminative and allays the possible griping of the laxative Senna.

Notes: Powdered Fennel enters into our effective Flea Powder for animals, large and small, and this formula we have prepared in our pharmacy for several years. Mix together 3 ounces each of powdered Fennel and Pyrethrum flowers (generally called "insect flowers" or powder) and one ounce of powdered Sassafras Bark.

For ants, mix the above formula with ½ quantity each of Borax and red Pepper. Mix and spread.

Don't forget to mix a few Fennel seeds in with your bird's food.

"He who sees Fennel and gathers it not is not a man, but a devil." *Physicians of Myddrai.*

FIG

Taken in moderation, this is an excellent article of food, wholesome and most nutritive. Be sure to buy only the unsulfured kind. Eat Figs principally with other sweet fruits, as Bananas and Dates, or Apples, Grapes and Avocado which are second best, but *not* with starches or proteins. Dr. Esser believes, too, that this wholesome fruit, which offers us its "rich and melting honeyed sweetness," is like the Date, an excellent replacement for store-bought candies. Says the doctor: "Instead of parents giving children candy that robs the vital minerals from their little bodies, they would be saving their children dental decay and other illnesses, if they were to substitute the wholesome fig, and other sweet fruits for unhealthful sweets. Not only is it a healthful food, but unlike other foods usually urged for children, it is one that is most appealing to and liked by all children."

As for its medicinal properties, it is an excellent nutritive as stated above. It may also be considered a laxative in habitual constipation and therefore must be eaten in moderation, for over-eating of this food may also produce undesired flatulence and even diarrhea. And its other therapeutics have been much employed for hundreds of years, just as they are today. One medical practitioner observed that Figs were a "useful ingredient in medicines intended for disorders of the chest, and in applying electuaries. Applied externally, either by themselves or in conjunction with other ingredients of a similar nature, they greatly forward the suppuration, or ripening of inflammatory tumors (boils)." And thus this old English proverb:

> Fig-poultice will our bodies rid of tumors,
> Scrofula, boils and even peccant humors;
> 'T will surely draw—add poppy heads alone
> The splintered fragments from a broken bone.

It is interesting to note that this food was used as a remedy for boils by Hezekiah over 2400 years ago. (Isaiah 38:21). And ever since then the Fig has been held in high repute for this purpose. Split open and soaked a minute or so in warm water, it forms an excellent poultice for an external, inflammatory boil and abscess, and a local application to a gum boil.

The juice obtained by soaking or stewing Figs is said to be a remedy for a simple sore throat or cough, temporary constipation and disturbances of the digestive tract.

Decoction of Figs: Boil an ounce of Figs in a pint of hot water for 5 or 6 minutes. Cover until cool and drink (sip slowly) a half cupful night and morning. This decoction is intended as a demulcent syrup in catarrhal and pectoral affections.

Gargle of Figs: The ingredients are ½ ounce of Figs, ½ ounce of Mallow Root (or Malva, Marshmallow or Hollyhock), and a pint of milk. Boil the milk, add the Mallow and Figs previously cut into small pieces, and simmer down to ¾ amount. Use as an emollient gargle in sore throat.

Compound Decoction of Figs: In 2 pints of hot water, boil 2 ounces each of Figs, Raisins and Barley. After 15 minutes of boiling, add ½ ounce Licorice root and allow to infuse. When cold, stir and strain. In ½ cupful doses taken night and morning, this is a demulcent laxative.

❦   ❦   ❦

GARLIC

Excerpts from *"The Lowly Garlic Is Highly Esteemed,"*
A Radio Talk

Garlic has had a long and interesting history from time immemorial. According to the Talmud, in Baba Kama, the eating of Garlic served many purposes. It satiated hunger, it kept the body warm, it brightened up the face, it killed parasites in the body, it fostered love and removed jealousy. The Egyptians, however, worshipped it and the Romans gave it to their laborers to impart strength, and to their soldiers to excite courage. Their game cocks were also fed with Garlic previous to fighting.

The Hindus have used Garlic for the past 300 years. The early Egyptians and Hebrews considered Garlic a food endowed with divine properties—and so it is really. The Irish have used it for centuries for treating coughs, and Pliny, the Roman naturalist, attributed curative powers to Garlic in respiratory and tubercular ailments. The Latin and French people, and the Romans and Greeks, have realized its subtle flavor for centuries. Aristophanes, the ancient playwright, mentions it many times in his comedies.

When it comes to medicinal virtues that's where friend Garlic just beams forth in all his glory. No doubt, many of you have read newspaper ads that told of Garlic being made sociable, having been manufactured into tablets that were supposed to be "pleasant and chewable like candy." Similar ads had it that Garlic tablets were indicated in the symptoms of high blood pressure or if one were "dull, tired, nervous, dizzy and (victim of) involuntary naps." The ads went on to say, "Why be distressed needlessly when you can get the effective aid of Garlic for relief, without fear of offending with Garlic breath?"

One of the oldest uses for Garlic has been in the preparations of a syrup for bronchial coughs and spasms especially in asthma. I can still recollect seeing my herbalist grandfather preparing such a syrup made of Flaxseeds, Skunk Cabbage Roots and Garlic and how pleased he would be, how his eyes would twinkle, when the asthmatic after having taken of the remedy for a week or so would report back to Grandfather that he, the asthmatic, could breathe and work and sleep so very much better.

It is a very rare occurrence, indeed, to find a member of the past generation of Italian descent, who is afflicted with either asthma or tuberculosis or with gall bladder disorders. This is so because mainly his daily menu calls for Garlic and Olive Oil in at least two of his heavier meals. Thus may he consider himself a true follower and practitioner of the sagacious advice of Hippocrates "The Father of all Medicine," who thousands of years ago said, "Let food be your medicine."

It is a fact that Bulgaria, up until that madman Hitler took over that nation, led in proportion of all other European nations in centenarians, who lived in small villages or mountainous districts and led regular but rather primitive lives. Indeed, they attributed their longevity to the diet of fresh vegetables and fruits and daily doses of sour milk and Garlic.

It is claimed that a teaspoonful of Garlic mixed with a tablespoonful of olive oil or soy bean oil, taken at night will liven up the liver and so rejuvenate it that the skin of the body will glow with renewed activity and the general welfare will be improved. A poultice made of crushed Garlic will also cure poison ivy. Crush several kernels of Garlic, place it between the layers of gauze and apply on the sore spots for about 30 minutes. It is indeed a miracle vegetable!

If it does not agree with one at first, it should be eaten sparingly, but the energy derived from the use of it should urge anyone to continue. By eating it at night, you will offend no one. A good idea is to get all your friends to eat it too and then no one will notice the garlic odor!

Garlic, like the other members of his family, Onion, Leek and Chives, offers to you an excellent source of vitamin C and a fair amount of vitamins A, B, and G. It abounds in the minerals of sulfur, iron and calcium.

If you want to partake of gradual doses of our odoriferous friend, may I suggest your trying out this experiment which I've found successful for both my own family and for my friends. Separate a whole Garlic into the respective cloves (some 6 or 8) and plant in rich well-drained soil, or in such soil that is adapted for the growing of Onions. Soon enough the scallion-like tops have grown 6 to 8 inches high, high enough to be cut, and are ready to be collected. Cut close to the original clove—about one inch above the soil—and then you may use either as is, or mixed with other greens such as Celery, Lettuce or crisp uncooked Spinach. Also you may incorporate them with a cole slaw, although I prefer the open or Caesar-type salad. In either case, be sure to include Cress (either Water or Gardencress) and our very good friend Parsley. In cold salads, these two, Parsley and Cress, will do the honors in disguising quite effectively the possible odors of the Garlic oil. However, it is here recommended that wherever there are digestive disturbances or inflammation of the bowels or stomach, Garlic must not be eaten (nor Onion, Chives or Leeks). As Dr. Meyrick noted: "The use of it appears very improper in hot bilious constitutions, where there is already too great a degree of irritation, or where the juices are thin and acrimonious, and the viscera unsound, in which cases it is almost certain to occasion headaches, flatulence, thirst and a variety of feverish symptoms."

Actually, Garlic should always be considered a most valuable medicinal—both as a preventative against possible disease and then as a curative—when needed. Daily doses taken any way possible will help to fight diseases of the nose and respiratory tract. It has been recommended for persons with high blood pressure. It has, as I've said before, been much used as an asthma remedy, and as a worm syrup. But moreover, it is an excellent intestinal antiseptic and an especially good stimulant to the digestive system.

I have a note here that says: "The attack of almost continuous sneezing which held 21 year old Juanita Lollis in its grip for six days, ended today at 1 p.m. A diet of Garlic, which halted the seizure for several hours Sunday night, was resumed today in modified form. Her sneezing, which had been as rapid as 15 per minute, gradually subsided and finally ceased when the diet was resumed."

Another note states that "there is doubtless virtue in Garlic and Onions and many of their sweet-smelling sisters, and they may again come into medical use. The thoughts of recent years, that their virtue was due to their odor, are further discussed in a work of Professor B. P. Tokin. He states that the essential oils of these substances contain constituents that kill bacteria, protozoa, and even larger organisms like yeast cells and the eggs of certain lower animals. Experimental uses of these compounds are now being made in hospitals, particularly in the treatment of suppurative wounds."

The following is taken from a recent news report: "Biological chemists have discovered a new germ-killing chemical in the common Garlic, which is called allicin. It not only attacks types of germs which can be vanquished by penicillin but also others which so far have proved themselves immune to this new wonder drug (penicillin). What Science has not discovered only goes to prove what a lot of people have suspected all along, that Garlic's penetrating, potent and persistent flavor and odor ought to influence germs just as surely as it does people—but in a different way.

Allicin, it is reported by Dr. John H. Bailey, of the Winthrop Chemical Co., who isolated it from Garlic, attacks one of the commonest of all germs—the staphylococci that are found in boils and does this not by actually destroying them on contact like iodine or bichloride of mercury, but by limiting the bacteria's ability for further growth. It helps destroy the germ's oxygen metabolism just as a person may smother to death.

After such studies, Dr. Bailey finds that it takes 100 times as much allicin from Garlic to fight the germs developed in boils as it does for penicillin. If that's all there were to it, scientists wouldn't be much interested. But the big point to remember is that the garlic chemical's value lies in combatting some of the germs that penicillin won't touch. Such a germ is bacillus para-typhoid A, which creates a disease in man closely resembling typhoid fever.

Paratyphoid bacteria have several types and this germ family creates a complicated variety of ailments which often confuse medical diagnosis by physicians. Sometimes they cause symptoms like those of the usual summer complaints. On other occasions they produce face influenza or rheumatism or kidney complications. Any advance that allicin can make against Paratyphoid bacillus will be welcomed by the medical fraternity.

Garlic Aids Digestive Process: If you are nervous or dyspeptic, you will be interested in a recent issue of the *Review of Gastroenterology* which reports that Garlic and its concentrates soothe the innards and permit the victims of nervous indigestion and other mind-made digestive troubles to feel better.

❦   ❦   ❦

That Garlic is considered an effective remedy for baldness or bald spots is not new, having been so employed for centuries. Here are two methods of application:

1. Cut ⅓ of a clove and rub in the juice. Allow to dry, and an hour later, massage in a few drops of a mixture of Bay Rum and Olive Oil. Do this morning and night.

2. Prepare this Capillary Lotion by macerating two cloves, cut into small pieces, in a pint of 90% alcohol for two days. Strain and add a cupful of either (cut) roots or fresh flower-heads of Burdock. Allow to stand five days and strain. The head, said the creator of this formula, is to be sponged with the lotion every evening for a month, "being efficient to promote the growth of hair."

Prevention reports that at the District Oncological Dispensary, Kirovograd, D. M. Sergaiev and I. D. Leonov have used Garlic in the treatment of 194 cases of lip and mouth disorders. The Garlic was rubbed in a mortar to make a paste and the paste was put on sterile gauze which was kept on the affected lip for 8 to 12 hours. 93.2% of the cases reported complete healing of such disorders as hyperkeratosis (a horny swelling), leukoplakia (white spots frequently precancerous) and fissures and ulcers of the lip.

🌷   🌷   🌷

How To Eat Garlic and Keep Your Friends: A subscriber to *Health Culture* says he can get all the benefits of garlic without its unpleasant effects by cutting the bulb in two, lengthwise and crosswise, and swallowing the small particles with a large draught of water from a good-sized spoon. He takes this each morning followed by the juice of a lemon, and after an hour no odor is discernible.

🌷   🌷   🌷

SWEET GERANIUM

This is the common House Geranium, Sweet or Apple-Scented Geranium and is more often referred to as a Pelargonium. It is largely cultivated as a decorative potted plant and is perhaps, of all house plants, the most familiar and the easiest of culture. And, to quote Horticulturist Bailey: "If a window has just one plant, that will be a Geranium."

An original recipe for an herb tea is thus prepared: Grind up small portions of the dried rinds of Lemon, Orange and Tangerine and mix; of which take ½ teaspoonful and an equal amount of dried Sweet Geranium and prepare a tea in a cupful of water. While drinking the liquid chew thoroughly bits of the fruit rinds. This tea is a good alkalizer.

To prepare an herbal sachet or potpourri, use equal culinary portions of Marjoram, Lavender, Sweet Geranium, Rosemary or Thyme, plus the ground peels of the castaways, Orange, Lemon and Tangerine. By adding a few yellow Tansy buttons to this combination, an effective moth preventative is prepared.

A present day custom in England is that of attaching small silk bags of Sweet Geranium and Lavender (both home grown) on the backs of living room chairs. Evidently this not only presents a pleasant and comforting atmosphere for the visitor, it definitely says, "no trespassing" to all destructive moths and their friends and relatives.

From *Better Health with Culinary Herbs.*

🌷   🌷   🌷

GINGER

This spice, as with Cloves, Pepper, Mustard and Cinnamon, plus finely crushed pure Camphor, when incorporated into unsalted lard, goose grease, or chicken fat, will compose today, as in Grandfather's time, a medicated plasma applied externally for bronchial congestion. Some kitchen chemists have first allowed the spices to simmer slowly in warm spirits of Turpentine for ½ hour; the strained liquid, cooked, is mixed with the ointment base. The finished product is used as a counter-irritant in relieving irritations and congestion in colds and coughs due to colds.

Powdered Spices	Of each one teaspoonful
Powdered Camphor	¼ teaspoonful
Spirit of Turpentine	1 ounce
Ointment Base	4 ounces

Note: The medication will prove more effective if first rubbed well into the affected area and then covered with flannel. Acts similarly to Vicks Vapo Rub, Musterole, etc.

Ginger Vapor for Quinsy: The ingredients, ½ ounce of powdered Ginger and a pint of milk, are heated in a suitable vessel with a small neck: Let the vapor be received as hot as can be endured with open mouth. Use as an inhalation. This formula was also known as Dr. Fuller's Vapour for Quinsy. "This euporiston," said that learned physician, "more powerfully than any gargle whatsoever, attenuates, melts down and draws forth, tough phlegm; which by obstructing the glands and spongy flesh and hindering the full passage of blood and humours through them, occasions the inflammation and tumour; and therefore, it more effectually takes off this perilous distemper than any of them."

Ginger Infusion: Macerate a teaspoonful of ground Ginger in a pint of hot water contained in a closed vessel. Allow to so remain for a half hour, stirring occasionally, and strain. A wineglassful dose taken warm or mixed with a little warm water every hour—or so as needed—will help to relieve menstrual cramps and discomfort, early symptoms of feverish colds and minor diarrhea complaints.

Ginger Lozenges: Use the above infusion and prepare lozenges as directed under Sugar.

Spice Plaster: Mix together 2 ounces of powdered Ginger and Cloves, 1 ounce of Cinnamon and 2 teaspoonsful of Red Pepper, incorporate ½ ounce of rubbing alcohol and allow the mixture to rest a half hour. Then mix in enough Honey to make the proper consistency for a stiff cataplasm.

Ginger Beer: In wineglassful doses, taken with hot water, it is intended as a valuable aid in the conditions listed under Ginger Infusion. It is to be prepared by a conventional formula which should, however, include Brown Sugar, Lemon and Honey.

GOOSE GREASE (GOOSE FAT)

See under Lard and Ointment Bases.

GRAPE, *the queen of fruits*

The juice of Grapes, freshly extracted, is a good blood fortifier and far better a source of quick energy than vitamin tablets or caffeine-bearing beverages. Do not, however, delude yourself by thinking that to gorge one's system with Grapes will eliminate the causes of your organic ailments. I am not an advocate of the so-called Grape-cure nor of any other food or drug cure, for neither is capable of producing a cure. But Grapes do help the body get rid of its accumulated toxins. "People of the Orient and Gandhi," said Dr. Floyd Bliss, "praised their use as a means of cleansing the inside of the body—and sometimes with startling results."

On the other hand, fresh Grape juice is easily assimilated and is indicated in poor appetite, constipation, gout and rheumatism, skin and liver disorders. This alkaline fruit helps greatly to decrease the acidity of the uric acid and lends itself further in aiding the elimination of the acid from the system, thus benefitting kidney function immensely.

As for food values, Grapes offer much of Vitamins A, B, and C, (Prof. Agamian believed that very little of C is contained in the green Grape) and appreciable percentages of the minerals sulfur, phosphorus, potassium and magnesium. Tartaric acid or more often, potassium acid tartrate, greatly abounds in the darker varieties of Grapes, and unlike the chemical as it appears in commerce, enhances the diuretic action. *Eat grapes alone;* with other foods, they may cause fermentation and digestive disorders. Although Grapes and the juice of Grapes are well tolerated and are digested most readily, they are not low in caloric content. Let the reducer beware for the over-consumption of either will add and not reduce needless weight.

❦   ❦   ❦

GRAPEFRUIT

Although the rinds of this fruit and those of its citrus cousins, Orange, Lemon and Tangerine, are usually discarded as worthless, they should be carefully dried, cut and grated, and saved for use in the winter months.

A level teaspoonful of the grated Grapefruit rind offers its benefits as a cold breaker remedy when steeped in a cup of hot water, either alone or with equal portions of Sage, Boneset and Mint. The dose is a warm cupful of the freshly prepared infusion every hour until desired results are obtained. Grapefruit is therefore called by some the fruit quinine.

By saving also the numerous seeds for immediate culture, one may realize further enjoyment of this worthy, health-sustaining fruit. The procedure is quite simple: Wash the seeds in cold running water and dry the excess water with a cloth. Then plant the seeds in vermiculite or a mixture of sand and soil (equal portions). Be sure that they are constantly watered. When seedlings are about 2 inches high, transplant into separate pots containing ⅔ sand, ⅓ soil.

The following is quoted from an advertisement which appeared in the newspapers (March 1959): "KEEP YOUR VITALITY UP! FIGHT COLDS WITH FRESH GRAPEFRUIT!

"To help keep colds and flu away, enjoy fresh Grapefruit from Florida at least twice a day. Grapefruit is rich in natural Vitamin C, one vitamin you need daily because your body cannot store it up.

"And it's important to get your Vitamin C—as nature intended—in combination with the other vital nutrients and health benefits in fresh grapefruit from Florida. That's what's meant by Vitality Vitamin C. For example, grapefruit and fresh-squeezed grapefruit provide other important vitamins and minerals. They provide energy from natural fruit sugars, extra liquids and help maintain alkaline reserve. All to help fight colds." *Florida Citrus Commission.*

Note: Eating Grapefruit may help fight Colds but living hygienically each and every day prevents far better the causes that lead to colds. (See under Lemon.)

"The fever is Nature's method of burning out poisons that would kill the body if they were not destroyed".

Harry Benjamin.

HONEY, *the king of sweets*

It is an accepted fact that Honey has long been recognized as a medicinal aid to more effectively soothe the irritation of a cough or sore throat. It is taken alone, i.e., as is, or diluted in warm water and a little Lemon juice, or as an ingredient in or as the sweetening agent of herbal cough syrups. Taken alone or diluted with an equal portion of water, a teaspoonful of Honey should be sipped slowly every hour and alternated with a dose of cough remedy every other hour. To relieve painful spasms of bronchial asthma, the following recipe, so an 88 year young herbalist informed me, has helped many a suffering asthmatic and may be prepared in one's kitchen laboratory: Half an Onion and two cloves of Garlic are simmered half an hour in a pint of Irish Moss jelly and when cool the mixture is strained through a sieve. To a pint of the strained jelly add half a cup of Honey, although true Maple Syrup or Molasses may be substituted for the Honey. The dose is a tablespoonful every two hours, sipped slowly alternating with Honey as previously mentioned.

A most pertinent feature of Honey is its germ-killing effects, claims Marc Dixon in *Honey—Food for Life and Health.* The distributors state, in advertising this book, that because of its hygroscopic and water-attracting properties, Honey has been found to be an invaluable dressing for wounds and burns. In one case cited in this book, a man found burned head to toe with scalding water, came out of his ordeal without a scar, and suffered little pain when Honey packs were placed on his wounds. Disease-producing germs cannot live without water, and it is due to this wonderful quality of absorbing water that makes Honey an excellent bacteria-killer. Tests have shown that a number of the worst disease-producing organisms have died when they came into contact with Honey.

A New Use for Honey

Honey has a very distinct bactericidal power which is mainly due to its moisture absorbing ability. All living micro-organisms require a certain amount of moisture to maintain their lives. When these micro-organisms come into contact with honey they are deprived of this much needed moisture and perish. Honey is acid in reaction which makes it an unfavorable medium for the micro-organisms to grow in. Micro-organisms which are harmful to the human body are destroyed in honey.

The moisture attracting ability of honey can be put to various uses. One of these is to attract and hold fluid in the child's body during the hours of sleep so that wetting of the bed will not take place. If a child is given honey, the blood and tissue calcium begins to increase. The calcium as it increases will unite with the excess phosphorus to form a compound that makes bones, teeth, hair and fingernails. It requires 2½ hours after taking honey for the blood and tissue calcium to rise in the adult body to the point where a check up of the blood phosphorus level shows that it has been lowered by uniting with the increased blood and tissue calcium. But the sedative effect on the nervous system of a child may be observed within an hour.

Honey does not require the process of human digestion before it is ready to enter the blood stream. It is in the blood stream within a half hour after it is taken. This explains in part the rapid sedative action on the body.

At bedtime the child is given a teaspoonful of honey. This will act in two ways. First, it will act as a sedative to the child's nervous system. Second, it will attract and hold fluid in the child's body during the hours of sleeping. By attracting and holding fluid, it spares the kidneys with the result that the child does not wet the bed during the night.

Experiment by omitting the honey at bedtime in order to learn if it is not possible to restore normal bladder control. You will soon begin to recognize the safe and unsafe nights as you study your child and the amount of its fluid intake especially after 5 o'clock. *J. C. Jarvis, M. D.*

According to a news report, an amazingly effective remedy for erysipelas is to cover the affected area generously with Honey. Cover well and a little beyond the affected area, then cover the Honey with cotton. Let remain for 24 hours. If necessary, repeat. "The above has never been known to fail among my family and friends."—*(E.H.)*

As an application to indolent ulcers, the following formula may be prepared: Yellow Wax, 1 ounce and Honey, 4 ounces. Melt the wax and slowly add the Honey, stirring well. Apply twice a day and bandage.

Mel Rose is the druggist's former preparation of Extract of Rose and Honey, etc., a mild astringent used as a gargle and mouth-wash and is of benefit as a douche, to relieve the inflammation of the mucous membranes of the nasal passages.

The *Oxymel* which was composed of one part each of Honey, Vinegar (acetic acid) and water, was once a popular gargle.

Honey mixed with glycerin and your favorite hand lotion will prove most serviceable as an emollient for chapped hands, irritated skin, etc.

🌰   🌰   🌰

HORSERADISH

The old-fashioned idea of a Spring tonic frequently calls for use of Horseradish. And to an epicure, Horseradish means more than just sauce for steak, or a concoction for an oyster dip. Horseradish has been employed as a food and medicine since the earliest days. It was first considered to be one of the bitter herbs—chrane and charosis, eaten by the Hebrews of Ancient Egypt during the Feast of Passover. (ED. The other four are Coriander, Horehound, Lettuce and Nettle.) The herbalists used it as a cough remedy and worm expellant. Some 350 years ago, Herbalist Gerard wrote: "The Horseradish stamped with a little vinegar put thereto, is commonly used for sauce to eat fish with and such like meates as we do mustard."

The chemical properties are similar to that of black Mustard. The active principle is singarin, producing a volatile oil known as allyl isothiocyanate.

Since the root serves in a dual capacity as a culinary edible, as do its cousins, Watercress, Wild Mustards and Nasturtium and others, the root may be sliced in transverse sections and served with oily fish and fatty meats. It may either be eaten by itself or seasoned lightly with oil, Lemon juice, or cider vinegar, but not with white vinegar which will prove harmful to the delicate mucous membranes of the stomach. Be sure to thoroughly masticate even the thinnest slice of Horseradish, that it may best furnish its warming stimulation to the digestive system. A gourmet acquaintance suggests to the neophytes undertaking the first few bites of this coarse root, to immerse several thin strips (cut lengthwise) of the well bruised root in white wine, add a few dried rinds each of Lemon and Orange, and allow to steep for about an hour before serving. M-m-m?

Fresh Horseradish root is richer in Vitamin C than Lettuce and Green Peppers.

There are many references to the therapeutics of Horseradish in medical compendia. It was officially accepted in the *United States Pharmacopoeia* (and *United States Dispensatory*) in the mid-1800's and until recently in the *British Pharmacopoeia* where it appeared together with Nutmeg and Bitter Orange Peel in the formula of Compound Spirit of Horseradish. Its many properties—stomachic and appetizer, stimulant to digestion, rubefacient, antiseptic, diuretic and antiscorbutic (anti-scurvy)—justify its well-deserved recognition in the above authoritative volumes as well as in the *French Codex* where it appears in the Compound Syrup of Raifort (Horseradish), formerly called Antiscorbutic Syrup.

All the better to corroborate the intensive research and closely observed findings by the medical, herb-minded physicians of an era preceding the publications of these compendia. Dr. W. Withering: "It is of a warm, stimulating diuretic nature, and often proves serviceable in paralytic and dropsical complaints." Dr. William Meyrick: "It is an excellent medicine in rheumatic complaints, and such as arise from obstructions of the viscera. It is likewise a powerful diuretic and frequently brings away small stones and gravel. Few things strengthen the stomach and assist digestion more than the root of this plant; and there is no better way of taking it than as it is commonly used at the table. It is likewise recommended in scorbutic complaints." Mr. W. Coles: "Of all things given to children for worms Horseradish is not the least, for it killeth and expelleth them."

I find this remedy for dropsy: An ounce of Horseradish root and ½ ounce of crushed Mustard seeds are steeped in a pint of hot water for 15-20 minutes. A cupful is drunk 3-4 times a day. A syrup may also be prepared and although originally intended for hoarseness and colds, doubles as an effective worm expeller.

Dr. Pope believes that a half teaspoonful flavored with a little Lemon juice should be taken twice a day morning and midafternoon, to help "dissolve the mucous in the sinus cavities and other parts of the body without damage to the mucous membranes. It acts as a solvent and cleanser of abnormal mucus in the human system."

IRISH MOSS

Irish Moss is generally considered the basic ingredient of many nutritive puddings and jellies and offers the much needed sulfur and iodine food elements to the human body, ill or well. It should likewise be considered a must kitchen remedy for a variety of ailments. Steeped in a warm pekoe tea solution, elsewhere mentioned, and strained when cool, the Moss yields a jelly that quickly soothes and heals a fresh burn or scalding, sunburn, etc.

Mixed with Cucumber juice and/or Quince seed jelly, Irish Moss offers a soothing hand lotion to apply to chafed or winter-chapped skin, although by far, it is much more employed as an excellent demulcent and emollient to allay stubborn coughs due to colds, in which case Honey and Lemon juice should be mixed with the Moss jelly.

Irish Moss Hand Lotion

Irish Moss	1 teaspoonful
Tragacanth flakes	1 teaspoonful
Borax	1 teaspoonful
Glycerin	1 ounce
Alcohol (Rubbing)	1 ounce
Water—enough to make a pint.	

Directions: Mix the Irish Moss and Tragacanth in a pint of boiling water and allow to stand until cool. Strain and add, in small amounts, the borax previously dissolved in a little water, and last, the glycerin and alcohol. Shake well.

If the preparation is intended to soothe winter-cracked or severely irritated skin, two teaspoonsful (¼ ounce) of Tincture Benzoin Compound are to be added to a pint of finished product. Be sure to add the Tincture in small amounts, about ¼ teaspoonful at a time, and shake vigorously after each addition.

A simple cough remedy may be prepared by boiling for a half hour a tablespoonful each of Boneset and Hoarhound in a pint of hot water, straining the mixture and adding a level tablespoonful of Irish Moss to the liquid. The resultant jell liquid is again strained and to it is added half a cup of Honey or brown sugar.

🌱　　🌱　　🌱

"The fruit thereof shall be for meat, and the leaf for medicine."   *Ezekiel* 47:12.

🌱　　🌱　　🌱

LANOLIN

Lanolin, also known as wool fat, is a very old medicament and is mentioned in the writings of Ovid, Pliny and Herodotus. It is much used today in medicine in chronic skin diseases where there is skin infiltration and where a penetrating action is desired. Lanolin has several advantages over lard and vaseline: It absorbs an appreciable amount of water, as Boric Acid Solution, it does not become rancid under ordinary conditions and its stickiness enables it to adhere quite tenaciously to the skin, being less liable to be washed off.

If necessary, lanolin may be cut down with lard or cooking oil (Cottonseed, etc.). When the active ingredient is a chemical like boric acid, zinc oxide, precipitated sulfur, first mix it well with a little mineral or cooking oil and then incorporate it with the lanolin.

Ointment Base: Dissolve together a heaping teaspoonful each of lanolin and beeswax and 3 ounces of petroleum jelly (or vaseline). A heavier base requires a larger amount of lanolin. The ointment base is described as an emollient and is often used as a mild dressing to blistered and bruised surfaces. And frequently it serves as a vehicle for other ointments.

Cod Liver Oil Ointment: Mix together 2 parts of Lanolin with 1 of the oil and then with 1 part of petroleum jelly (petrolatum) or vaseline. Use as a dressing for burns, sunburn, etc.

Benzoin Ointment: Stir together ⅓ teaspoonful Tincture Benzoin Compound and a teaspoonful of petrolatum; then incorporate with an ounce of lanolin. This ointment is indicated in irritations of the skin, cuts, etc. (See under Tincture Benzoin Compound).

❦ ❦ ❦

LARD

This is a very handy ointment base in which to administer powdered spices as Cloves, Pepper, Mustard and others. Remember to mix the powder first in a little Olive Oil and then into the base. If the skin ailment is merely superficial, the lard base may be "stretched out" with an equal amount of petroleum jelly.

In the absence of lard, the following may be substituted: Butter, chicken fat, cold cream, goose grease, hydrogenated vegetable oils as Spry and Crisco and mutton suet.

❦ ❦ ❦

LEEK

The Leek, the national emblem of the Welsh, grows wild in Switzerland but here, as in many countries, it is cultivated as a vegetable and seasoning herb. It is another shining example of an herb-vegetable's offering its services as a mouthful of *preventative medicine*. Leeks should be served as a greens replacement for Chives, Scallions, and Onion and Garlic tops.

Be sure to eat the alkaline-forming greens *uncooked* and to *chew them well*.

The therapeutic properties resemble those of Onion, Garlic, et al, for the active principle of these foods is the volatile oil

containing allyl sulfide. It is the oil that gives to all parts of
the plant the characteristic mildly acrid taste and gently pungent odor. Its action is noted by the *United States Dispensatory* as "generally stimulant, with a direction to the kidneys.
The dose of the expressed juice is about a teaspoonful." This
advice recalls that of a prominent medical practitioner of the
late 18th century: "The juice of Leeks is a good diuretic and
will frequently afford relief in the stone and gravel, when
most of the usual remedies fail." This reference to Herbalist
Hill's recommendation of its further medicinal values is noted:
"An infusion of the roots boiled into a syrup with honey, is
a good medicine in coughs, asthma and disorders of the breast
and lungs. It answers the same purpose with syrup of Garlic,
but being milder and not so strong, it may be taken by many
who cannot bear that medicine."

LEMON

This fine, tart fruit has long been known for its excellent
antiscorbutic (anti-scurvy) properties. Up to several years ago,
English law required sailing ships to carry enough Lemon or
Lime juice so that, after being 10 days at sea, each sailor
would receive his daily minimum of one ounce. But, if one
is to benefit from the food values, both vitamins and minerals,
it is important to eat at least one thin slice of this very good
food a day—unsweetened. "The highly acid taste," states Dr.
Esser, "that at first calls forth the saliva in great amounts and
screws up the face, is only an experience that goes with the
first or second Lemon one eats. After a few tries, eating a
Lemon as it is becomes a delightful and refreshing experience."

The Lemon is a very rich source of Vitamins B, C, P and
riboflavin, and of minerals calcium, phosphorus, magnesium,
potassium and sulfur.

As for its medicinal virtues, we find that in Elizabethan
days, in the British Isles and America, the outermost rind or
peel of Lemons was considered a "grateful aromatic and an
excellent ingredient of infusions intended to strengthen the
stomach. The juice made into a Syrup is excellent to be taken
in fevers. It is likewise used—as a gargle for inflammations of

the mouth and throat. Joined with a small quantity of Cinnamon, it generally puts a stop to those severe vomitings that sometimes happen in fevers."

We find that some herbalists recommend a combination of Lemon peels, Gentian root and Sassafras bark to increase the power of stomachics. Some herbalists also advise us to boil the spongy portions of the rind in water, to evaporate the decoction, and thus to obtain pure crystals of *hesperidin* which are readily deposited.

We find also that Lemon and its juice are valuable therapeutic aids as a diuretic in rheumatism and as a quick-acting diaphoretic and anti-periodic (temperature reducer) in feverish colds. A little of the juice mixed with a little warm water (or Sage tea) and Honey yields a healing astringency of service as a gargle for sore throat.

Lemon has its external applications as well. For acne and blackheads rub the juice directly on to the affected area and allow to dry; or apply a mixture of equal parts of the juice and Rose Water (prepared by steeping a few Rose Petals in hot water). In either case, apply morning and night. As a face and freckle bleach, I have prepared a cream of a tablespoonful of equal parts of Lemon Juice and Rose Water in which is mixed enough powdered Elder flowers to make a paste. And this is incorporated in enough cold cream to yield 2 oz.

Remember that the juice also is highly prized as an after-shampoo rinse, to invigorate the scalp and hair. For dandruff, massage the scalp with a little juice and allow to dry, before shampooing.

🌿　🌿　🌿

Discover New Key to Health and Vigor

Discovery of a new key to human health and vigor, through studies of a chemical extracted from Lemon peel, was revealed. In the light of this discovery, it appears that the spongy rind of Lemon skins contains the raw material of an important agent of health.

Previous investigations made by Professor Szent-Georgyi, Nobel Prize winner and noted Hungarian medical scientist, and other biochemists have led to the assumption that lemon peels contain a peculiar vitamin called "Vitamin P," which aids in preventing rupture and weakness of capillary blood vessels.

Thus, this supposed vitamin plays a part of its own, different from that of Vitamin C, in preventing bleeding due to easy breaking of the walls of fine blood vessels.   *G. B. Lal.*

"Blood" Made from Skin of Citrus Fruits

Discovery of an "artificial blood" derived from citrus fruit pectin was announced today by physicians in the Henry Ford Hospital laboratories.

Vital to warring nations, the discovery is expected to supplant blood transfusions in treatment of shock. The pectin is easily and inexpensively prepared from the skins of the ordinary lemon or grapefruit. The pectin has been used successfully on 25 hospital patients. Dr. Hartman said British authorities have consulted him regarding the discovery. He said the "blood" could be bottled and stored at room temperature.   *News Report.*

The Herbalist Almanac says that lemon seeds if planted and treated as house plants, will make pretty little shrubs. The leaves can then be used for flavoring. Tie a few lemon leaves in a piece of muslin or cheesecloth and drop in apple sauce when boiling and nearly done. It is an inexpensive way to flavor the sauce.

The hands may be made soft and supple by daily applications of fresh lemon juice. Rubbing around nails and cuticle with lemon juice daily keeps those areas in good order.

I do this morning, noon, and night—It makes my nails so nice and white! Good beauty hint, Petunia! Rub your fingernails with a bit of lemon peel regularly and it will whiten them and strengthen them too.   *News Column.*

🌷   🌷   🌷

MARIGOLD

Part Used: The flower heads and florets, collected when fully expanded and carefully and quickly dried, away from the sunlight.

This is the common Pot or Garden Marigold that is grown in flower gardens as a mere do-nothing ornament, its many benefits unfortunately not at all utilized. At the beginning of the century, this worthy herb (then called by its Latin name *Calendula*) was cultivated in the herb or kitchen garden and, as were also Witch Hazel (*Hamemelis*) and Barberry (*Barberis*) and others, extensively used by the prudent and enterprising kitcheneer as seasoner, dye and medicine.

Season and color your next rice or cheese pudding with a mild sprinkling of the flowers. They'll do well in your baking bread, cookies or pastry. As recently as 25 years ago, farm folk churned the petals with the cream to dye the butter yellow.

Dr. Meyrick quotes his contemporary, practitioner Dr. Hill, "An infusion of the fresh gathered flower is good in fevers. It gently promotes perspiration and throws out anything that (symptomatically) ought to appear on the skin." And he states that as a result of much observation, "a water distilled from them (the freshly gathered flower-heads) is good for inflamed and sore eyes. A decoction of the flowers in posset drink is much used among country people as an expulsive in the smallpox and measles." Before Dr. Meyrick's time, the writers and physicians recommended a solution of the flowers as an eye drop for "red and watery eyes," and would "cease the inflammation and taketh away the pain"; while a syrup of the flowers was said to "cure the trembling heart."

Today, though not much employed by the herbalist, the petals of Marigold are incorporated into *Calendula Cream*, a soothing, healing salve, which is today manufactured by the Otis Clapp Co. of Boston. And an application for cuts and bruises is easily made by the kitchen chemist by steeping 2 teaspoonsful of the petals in 2 ounces of ethyl rubbing alcohol. Allow to steep 10 days, stir and strain through absorbent cotton. Or if an ointment is desired, slowly simmer for 10 minutes a tablespoonful of the petals in about 4 ounces of unsalted lard, strain through cheese cloth and store in the refrigerator.

A cosmetic astringent or skin cleanser may be thus prepared: Steep for a week a few flower heads in *enough* Witch Hazel to cover, stir and strain; or simmer gently for 5-6 minutes one teaspoonful of dried ground petals in 4 ounces of cold cream.

Herbalist Turner wrote, 1568: "Some use it to make their

heyre (Hair) yellow with the flour of this herbe not being content with the natural color which God hath gyven them."

❦   ❦   ❦

MARJORAM

Marjoram is an all purpose herb, will delightfully season almost all foods and being one of many kitchen medicines, serves in other capacities. Long before Hops entered the preparation of ales and wines, Marjoram imparted its own characteristic "grand taste" to these home-made brews. And the many centuries that have witnessed the use of the herb in the manufacture of cosmetics and perfumes have also noted its equally outstanding property as a source of many therapeutic values.

John Gerard informs us that he and his herbalist contemporaries signified Sweet Marjoram as a "remedy against cold diseases of the brain and head (dizziness or headache). . . . It easeth the tooth-ache being chewed in the mouth. . . . The leaves boiled in water, and the decoction drunk easeth such as are given to overmuch sighing. . . . The leaves dried and mingled with honey put away black and blue marks after stripes and bruises, being applied thereto. The leaves are excellently good to be put into all odoriferous ointments, water, powder, broths and meats. . . . There is an excellent oyle to be drawn forth from these herbes, good against the shrinking of sinus, cramps, convulsions, and all aches proceeding of a cold cause." Many of these old-time uses are quite as applicable in this day of skepticism, only we moderns find that the aforementioned preparations are today called, as sold by the druggist, liniments, counter-irritants, analgesic balms, spirits, antacids, carminatives, etc.

And in John Parkinson's statement (1629), "Marjoram herb is used in meats and broths to give relish unto them and to help a cold stomach and to expel wind," do we find the basic reason why culinary herbs must be added to all prepared foods: Yes, to delicately season cooked or prepared foods, the better to digest their nutrients and most important, to prevent unforeseen illness.

The camphoraceous principle contained in the leaf oil causes Marjoram to be employed as a medicinal.

Headache or nervousness: Mix equal parts of Marjoram, Sage, Catnip and Peppermint and a warm tisane (of the mixture one teaspoonful is steeped for 5-6 minutes in a cup of hot water) is sipped *slowly* every hour or two until relieved. Minus the Sage, the mixture is of good service as a remedy for indigestion, stomach upset, nausea, etc.

Measles: Steep ⅓ teaspoonful each of Marjoram, Yarrow and Catnip (plus a pinch of Saffron or Marigold or Safflower) to prepare a tisane. The warm tea given to the reluctant patient every hour will hasten the eruption, the better to overcome and dispel the attending fever.

❦ ❦ ❦

"Overweight is not a joke. It is a definite disease as deadly as any to be found in medical dictionaries."

Eugene Christian.

❦ ❦ ❦

MILK

Here is a portion of a letter from one of my radio program listeners who was a beginner in herb usage and could not say "honestly" that she did "enjoy herb tea." "I have formed," she wrote, "the bad habit of wanting a snack before retiring so I tried something new for a warm drink. I put some dry Sage leaves in cold milk, heated, but not boiled it, then covered it. I let it stand until it was cool enough to drink," wrote Mrs. T. J. H.

Others have reported to me that drinking warm milk before retiring has a most soothing and sedative effect upon the nervous system, being at times beneficial in inducing a more restful sleep.

Milk may be used as a wet compress to give temporary relief of acute sores.

Mrs. Thomas Healey: "An eye burn or irritation due to accidental access by table salt or a spice as Pepper or Mustard may be quickly remedied by inserting one or two drops in each corner of the eye."

Grandfather: "A simple home remedy that relieves an irritating cough may be made by mixing a teaspoonful each of

Honey and oil of Sesame in a cup of warm milk and sipping it slowly, until the mixture is all taken."

For a milk and bread poultice, see under Bread.

Drink no milk (or water or other fluids) with your meal. DRINK IT ALONE OR LEAVE IT ALONE.

"Milk soured by bacteria is considered a healthy drink. The *acidophilus* bacillus and the bacillus *bulgaricus* contained in such milk, counteract other germs which cause intestinal putrefaction."

Diarrhea Remedy for children: Warm a cup of milk and add 2 or 3 pinches or about 1/16 of a teaspoonful of powdered Cinnamon. For adults, use double amount of Cinnamon.

Nature's milk! In Peru the cow tree has sap which is sweet and nourishing milk.   *V.N.D.*

❦   ❦   ❦

MINERAL OIL

The use of mineral oil for any but external purposes is to be strongly discouraged. It has been the chief ingredient in commercial nose drops and laxatives and fortunately for the consumer, the use of this oil has gone the way of so many other chemical drugs, to its final resting place in the therapeutic limbo. As if to remind us of its past unsavory reputation, *The Dispensatory* warns us that "the direct instillation of (liquid) petrolatum in the nostril is not without danger, especially in children; cases have been reported in which *the oil trickled into the bronchi and caused pneumonia.*"*

Mineral oil, or any proprietary containing the oil, should not be used as nose drops, for in most cases, they do not give even relief to the nasal passages. Dr. Loeb has written that they "have absolutely no value in either preventing or curing a cold." And furthermore, he tells us, when either ephedrine, Pine oil, menthol or other aromatic principle is combined with the oil, there is a "sign of temporary relief due to the odor or astringent action of the drugs, but *more often the careless use of nose drops has carried a localized infection into the sinuses.*"*

Do not use the oil as a laxative or as an intestinal lubricant. There are two well documented objections against the use of

---

* My italics.

mineral oil for internal purposes, and here again *The Dispensatory* gives corroborative evidence: "A possible interference with intestinal absorption *and the fear based upon the known carcinogenic effects of the crude oil that it might give rise to cancer of the bowels.*"* It notably lessens the absorp-

* My italics.

tion of the Vitamin A and perhaps also D, presumably because of its solvent effect towards these vitamins. To which Dr. J. C. Molner, representing the views of the American Medical Association in a syndicated column attests that the oil will absorb Vitamin A and can prevent you from obtaining the vitamin *in the food you eat.**

Mineral oil may be used to "prepare" chemical or herbal ingredients before mixing them into the solid ointment base. For instance, the zinc oxide and Corn Starch (which see) of Lassar's paste are first mixed with a little of the oil to form a smooth mixture before being incorporated with the solid petrolatum (vaseline).

Players of stringed instruments consider the oil valuable in keeping their violins or cellos free of the ever-accumulating rosin. A few drops wiped over the instrument does the job quickly and effectively. I have always used a thin mineral oil to clean my viola.

❧ ❧ ❧

"God heals, and the Doctor takes the fee."

Benjamin Franklin.

❧ ❧ ❧

MOLASSES

Molasses has, in the past few years, been rediscovered as a quick energy food, a source of the vitamin B factors, plus the anti-anemia minerals of calcium, iron and potassium which help to prevent hardening of the arteries, etc. And too, Molasses has its place in medicine. It has already been mentioned as a substitute for Honey in cough syrups, etc. It is used in pharmacy as an excipient for pills and prevents hardening because of its hygroscopic, i.e., water absorbing, property.

* My italics.

This latter fact plus the claim that Molasses, Honey and other natural sugars, possess valuable antiseptic properties, recommends its use in the treatment of certain forms of wounds, infections and boils. For this purpose, a poultice is prepared with Molasses and ground, dark bread crumbs or flour, and applied to the affected area.

In feverish colds, an enema made of Molasses and Milk (one to four parts) has been given with good results. This is especially applicable to children and the aged.

🌷   🌷   🌷

MUSTARD

Prepared Mustard is not recommended as a seasoning agent, since the ingestion of the slightest excess may cause an unforgettable inflammation of the stomach and intestinal canal. The emetic effect is produced by the taking of one or two teaspoonful of the dry powder.

Flour and Mustard Poultice: Mustard, ground—1 tablespoonful, flour—3 tablespoonsful. Mix the powders intimately with an equal portion of warm water and vinegar. Of this recipe it was said that it was "beneficially employed to attract the blood from the deep seated or inward to the superficial or outward capillaries, or hair-like veins or arteries."

Even before the days of Hippocrates, the strongly pungent ground yellow Mustard has been in use for sufficient reason, as a counter-irritant.* For this purpose either of two methods of preparation may be used: 1. A heaping tablespoonful is mixed in a quart of boiling water and the thin mixture applied as a wash or by repeated wet applications. 2. A poultice may be prepared by mixing enough water with ½ to ⅔ cupful of powdered Mustard and this applied as a fomentation to the affected area.

Mustard for Musty Jars: You can remove odors from jars and bottles by following this suggestion: Pour a solution of water and dry mustard into the bottle and let stand for a few hours. Then rinse in hot water.

🌷   🌷   🌷

---

* Counter irritant: an agent intended to counteract or relieve pain or inflammation, by direct application.

Hot Mustard Foot Bath Eases Aches

Twenty years ago, I gave here instructions for administering (not taking, for you can't properly take it by yourself) a hot mustard foot bath and gave my opinion that it is the No. 1 first aid remedy for acute earache, acute alveolar abscess (ulcerated tooth), acute coryza, acute bronchitis, acute sinusitis or acute pneumonia.

The pain of acute earache, acute alveolar abscess or abscess at the root of a tooth, acute sinusitis, etc. is due to congestion and inflammation. The effect of the bath is to fill the surface vessels with blood, equalizing distribution of the blood and thus to relieve congestion or tension of blood in the ear, at the root of the tooth or in the sinus. One critic was annoyed because I said a hot mustard foot bath without a nurse to administer it is scarcely worth while. He asked whether a hot mustard ear bath would relieve toe ache. I had to admit the suggestion seemed feasible— at least for one with long ears. One of my first teachers when I was an intern routinely treated pneumonia with hot mustard foot baths—one every two hours in the early stage, less frequently after the first few days. I cannot recall that he ever lost a battle with pneumonia.   *Dr. William Brady.*

NUTMEG

The powdered spice has been considered a worthy aromatic carminative to remove flatulence, correct nausea arising from other drugs, and to allay vomiting. For either of these purposes, the dose is ⅛ to ¼ teaspoonful of the powder in a cup of water taken every hour until better. For simple diarrhea, a similar dose may be given.

In Grandfather's days, a compound containing Nutmeg was the druggist's Aromatic Powder which also contained Cinnamon, Ginger and Cardamon. This compound powder served not only as a quick-acting stomach remedy but especially as flavoring for cookies and pies.

OAT

A thin gruel prepared by boiling 1 ounce of Oatmeal in 3

pints of water until it measures a quart and pouring off the clear liquid from the sediment affords a nutritious bland aliment which is slightly laxative. (Cooked Oats mixed with Honey has been found of service in habitual constipation). This Oatmeal water may be sweetened with Honey which enhances its therapeutic quality and thus for bottle fed infants, it will be found to be a more effective laxative than Barley water. Ol' Doc Will Brady used to recommend that part of the water for the diluting of cow's Milk to modify it for feeding infants 5-6 months old, be replaced with strained Oatmeal water. Gradually, suggested the doctor, the Oatmeal water is to be replaced with thickened gruel and then unstrained Oatmeal so that in 3-4 months, the baby will go for a cereal gruel as well as for a ripe Banana.

During the Civil War, Oatmeal was made into a "common cake" baked and browned like coffee, then ground and made into an infusion, formed a drink that was "found excellent for nausea, dysentery, diarrhea, cholera morbus and irritable conditions of the stomach."

Oatmeal Poultice: To a cupful of meal add hot water and stir until it is sufficiently consistent. Or, mix one part of Oatmeal and 2 parts of Flax-seed and add enough hot water to prepare a thick poultice. Use as a cataplasm for bruises and open wounds.

Furacin, a yellow powder derived from the hulls of oats, appears to be another valuable new drug. Believed to be bactericidal as well as bacteriostatic, this nitrofuran has been used in the treatment of infected ulcers and superficial skin infections with "very good" results.

❧   ❧   ❧

"He is the best doctor who knows the worthlessness of most drugs."   *Sir William Osler.*

❧   ❧   ❧

OINTMENT BASES

Simple Ointment, as prepared by the druggist contains 5% each of Lanolin and Wax and 90% White Petrolatum (petroleum Jelly). It is described as an emollient and generally is used as a mild dressing to blistered or bruised surfaces. More frequently it serves as a vehicle for other ointments. Yet, any, or even a combination of the following articles, the majority of which almost every home possesses, may be employed as ointment bases: Butter, Chicken Fat, Cold Cream, Goose Grease, Hydrogenated Vegetable Oils (Spry, Crisco), Mutton Suet, Lanolin, Lard, Petrolatum Jelly (or Vaseline).

When using animal fats as a base in which powdered spices as Mustard and Pepper are to be incorporated, remember to first mix them with a little Olive Oil and then into the base. If petrolatum jelly (vaseline) is to be used, use mineral oil with which to mix the powder.

The hydrogenated oil will work as well as cold cream. When using lard, mix in 50% of Petroleum Jelly.

OKRA

This food was first introduced into the United States from Africa about 100 years ago, where it was known by its given name. The capsular fruit is a long ribbed pea which abounds in a mucilage called gombine. When green and tender, it may be included in salads, but generally it is added to gumbo-type soups or stews because of its especial thickening qualities. If not eaten uncooked, they may be steamed about 5 minutes in a very small amount of hot water.

Every part of the Okra may be engaged in several profitable ways and being quite mucilaginous and of a softening nature, may be employed wherever an emollient or demulcent is indicated. The leaves, Dr. Brown assures us, "make an unsurpassable relaxing (and healing) cataplasm." The extremely long roots and leaves contain much of the needed mucilage and have long replaced those of the scarce Marshmallow—to which they are said to be superior. After the fruits have been plucked, we have uprooted entire plants, washed them in cold water to remove any adhering soil, and after cutting the component parts, stems, leaves and roots into smaller segments and drying them in our attic, have used any of these parts as substitutes for Mallow or Marshmallow. (A fourth member of this group, Hollyhock, may be similarly treated.)

Any of the aforementioned parts should be employed whenever possible as a demulcent and emollient in the inflammation and irritation of the alimentary, respiratory, and urinary organs, in which case as much of Okra pods must be eaten as taste and disposition will permit. To use the leaves or roots, simmer a heaping tablespoonful of the dried, ground leaves or ½ tablespoonful of the roots in 2 pints of hot water, for 20 minutes or until only 1½ pints remain. Cover until cool, stir and strain. Drink the contents in equal amounts during the day.

To prepare a cough syrup, prepare with a teaspoonful of Flax-seeds and when strained add Honey, and to yield an asthmatic remedy, add a teaspoonful of freshly cut Onion; to prepare a diuretic remedy, add dried Corn Silk and Asparagus, (which see), a heaping teaspoonful of each to the Okra liquid.

Any part of these plants or herbs has the especial quality of healing an external sore or ulcer. I well recall the following incident: A diabetic friend whose leg ulcer would not respond to external applications of cortisone and other antibiotic ointments, finally after months of such fruitless treatment, applied a fresh clean leaf of Okra upon his leg ulcer 3 times a day for 2 weeks and then twice a day for another 2 weeks. During the last week, a thin slice of Onion was placed upon the Okra leaf and carefully bandaged. Another week of such poulticing and there were sure signs of recovery.

Blood "Plasma" Made from Pods of Okra: A Marquette University research team announced recently that they have been able to turn a common garden vegetable into a cheap and plentiful substitute for life-giving blood plasma. The plasma replacement is a product of okra pods.

The new material has all the advantages of blood plasma, it was said, and none of its disadvantages. It contains none of the harmful elements that can cause serious after-effects to recipients of human plasma in transfusions.

Also the plasma substitute can be obtained easily in powder form and less than an ounce of it makes up the equivalent of a quart of human plasma when a salt solution is added.

OLIVE OIL

The householder generally considers Olive Oil as a dressing

and salad oil for table use which, together with Garlic and Vinegar, is often used to season a salad of vegetables (subtly pre-seasoned by Nature). The pale-yellowish to green oil, commercially expressed from Olives, possesses one feature which makes it invaluable for food and medicine. It is non-volatile and non-drying. It is, therefore, much used for cooking purposes and alone is wholly nutritious. However, better than Olive are Soy, Corn and Peanut Oils, for they are far richer in the anti-cholesterol essential unsaturated fatty acids (or Vitamin F). From a nutritional point of view, the unsaturated fatty acids are quite essential since the body does not "manufacture" them. They are derived principally from cereal and vegetable oils (above mentioned) and from such foods as Nuts, Avocados and Sunflower seeds. But if they are to perform a better job of preventing cholesterol from being deposited in the blood-stream, *it is equally important to keep at a minimum all animal fat, butter, margarine, hydrogenated fats and shortenings, which are the main sources of the cholesterol.*

In industry it enters into the manufacture of hair preparations, toilet soaps, machine lubricants and illuminants. Its application as an ingredient in the Herbal Hair Tonic formula is mentioned under Castor Oil. The druggist's Sweet Oil is none other than Olive and is much used as a remedy for earache. (Castor Oil was formerly called Bitter Oil.) Warm and insert into ear a few drops, plug with cotton and apply hot water bottle.

Question: I wonder if you could tell me what I could do to a palm, and fern plant to pep them up. They have looked droopy for a couple of weeks—*Miss W.D.S.*

Answer: Two tablespoonsful of Olive Oil at the root of your palm or fern once a month will make a decided improvement in the plant.   *News Report.*

One of the writer's favorite pharmaceutical formulae is Caronol which is a soothing emulsion composed principally of Olive Oil and Lime Water and aromatics. It is intended to bring quick relief for fresh burns, sunburn and bed sores. As the name implies, this preparation is a revised form of the good old stand-by, Carron Oil, which the druggist prepares by mixing together equal parts of Linseed Oil and Lime

Water. Carron Oil is the name given to the latter preparation since it was first employed at the Carron Iron Works in Scotland and applied by the workmen for the relief of freshly acquired burns and scalds.

As previously stated, it is easily prepared by mixing thoroughly equal parts of Olive or Linseed oil and cold (chilled) lime water. And for best results, prepare this mixture only when needed and shake it well before using. It is applied to burns and acute inflammatory affections of the skin and thus serves as an excellent protective, coating the surface and excluding the air.

Olive Oil Massage Helped Bursitis

Dear Hopeful—I read your appeal for advice on bursitis of the shoulder. My husband had arthritis for seven years and at one time got a bad case of bursitis in his right shoulder and was unable to raise his arm. To relieve the soreness I started massaging the shoulder and upper arm daily with hot olive oil, using slight manipulation while massaging. This helped and gradually he got the motion back in his shoulder and hasn't been bothered with bursitis since.   *News Column.*

In medicine, it has been employed as a mild laxative (dose ½ to 2 ounces) in chronic constipation "especially when associated with malnutrition. . . . In the form of an enema, it is often a useful remedy in fecal impaction."

Medical doctors frequently have prescribed equal portions of Olive and Wintergreen oils as a liniment to relieve rheumatic pains. However, for best results, to the affected area there should first be applied several soaks of warm water and after the area is dried well, there is applied the aforementioned liniment.

Under Castor Oil, it has been suggested that it be used in a hair tonic preparation, plus added ingredients of Olive Oil, Alcohol, etc. The medical doctor often suggests to a patient with a dry, scaly scalp or dandruff the following procedure: The patient vigorously massages the scalp with a mixture of even parts of warmed Olive and Castor Oil until the scalp begins to tingle.

Oil Shampoo: To 3 ounces of Tincture Green Soap, add ½ ounce each of Castor and Olive Oils. Shake well before using and so label the bottle. Use tepid, *not* hot, water for the shampoo, and rinse with cold water (to which a little Lemon juice may be added).

(See under Camphor.)

Vegetable and Hydrogenated Oils. See under Ointment Bases.

ONION

"A syrup made of the juices of Onions and Honey, is an excellent medicine in asthmatic complaints." *Dr. Hill.*

Onions, when plentifully eaten, procure sleep, help digestion, cure acid belchings, remove obstructions of the viscera, increase the urinary secretions, and promote insensible perspiration. Steeped all night in spring water, the infusion given children to drink in the morning, while they are fasting, kills worms. Onions bruised with the addition of a little fat, and laid on fresh burns, draw out the fire, and prevent them from blistering. Their use is fitted to cold weather, and for aged, phlegmatic people, whose lungs are stuffed and their breath short. *From a letter, author unknown.*

One newspaper columnist (Albert Deutsch) some years ago, said:

For many centuries common, unschooled people in many lands have regarded the lowly onion as a healing agent. It has been used in the treatment of many ailments down the ages. It may be that medical science will soon provide scientific vindication for this 'grandmother remedy' in the treatment of burns and perhaps, as a general bacteria-killing agent. Medical history reveals many instances in which a scientific 'discovery' had been long known and applied by ordinary folk who never figured out why a thing worked, but knew that it did work. Many of the herbs now used as basic ingredients in standard medicines have been used as folk remedies for centuries.

As if that isn't sufficient proof of the versatility of friend Onion's values both as food and medicine, here are a few pointers from my little black notebook: "An Onion, dipped in

Honey and salt mixed with Hen grease (chicken fat), was used in the Middle Ages to remove red and blue spots from the complexion."

There is an old belief that the juice of an Onion rubbed into the scalp was good for curing baldness. When made into a soup, it was especially beneficial in infections of the nose and throat, and eaten as raw as possible during the late evening, is believed by many to aid the insomniac in sleeping.

Two members of our Herb Club report the following experience with friend Onion: Mrs. Adelia Frye was visiting her brother in Maine several months ago at a time when that gentleman was ailing with a stubborn and persistent cough. He had tried doctors and cough syrup and the usual run of patent remedies from the drug store, and every time he visited the physician or had bought another cough syrup, our heroine, Adelia, would needle him with, "Well, when are you going to stop wasting your money and your health and when are you going to take a simple remedy that I can make for you right here in the kitchen?" And, of course, the dear brother gave in finally and I cannot say whether it was because of his sister's needling or due to the severity of his ailment. However, as Mrs. Frye tells it, her brother said to her finally: "O.K., bring on your herbs and your Onion syrup. After all the other stuff I've taken, well—I'll bet you $5.00 that you can't cure this cough. Huh! you and your Onion syrup."

Undaunted was Mrs. Frye with her herbs and her Onion syrup. The Onion syrup prepared in a few minutes in the kitchen did not bring about any miraculous cure within an hour, but suffice it to say that hourly doses of the syrup begun by the reluctant brother in the morning, did bring great relief from the hacking and the coughing and pain and complaints. And this occurred before suppertime of that same day. Not only did sister Adelia win the $5.00 bet, but also her brother's promise never again to depend on patent medicines for the relief of a cough or other ailment, but rather on home-made remedies as herb and Onion syrup, or a hot tea of Catnip and Sage for feverish colds.

The other member of our Herb Club who told me of a medicinal use for the Onion is Mrs. T. J. Healy, authority on dyeing cloth with our native plants. Mrs. Healy's recounting of her Onion-experience runs something like this. It was during 1918, when the United States was embroiled in World

War I, and at that time, as many of us can well remember, the influenza epidemic was claiming as many casualties as did the battle fields. "But," says Mrs. Healy, "every day, three times a day, we had our bowls of strong onion soup. If any of us were sick several large sized onions were sliced transversely and placed in different parts of the sick room. It was my family's belief that small onion blisters had attracted and destroyed the virulent disease-causing germs. And, too, sliced onions constituted the greater portion of chest poultices."

Asthma Remedy (Source Unknown). Place very thin slices of raw Onion on a plate, spread Honey on each slice and cover with a plate. Allow to stand all night. Take a teaspoonful of the Honey 3 or 4 times a day, sipping slowly.

To brighten the gold leaf of your picture frames, it has been suggested to rub it with boiled Onion Juice, then wipe dry.

If you plant an Onion in the center of hills of Cucumbers, Melons, and Squash you will find that no worms or bugs will feed on these foods.

❦   ❦   ❦

ORANGE

John Harvey Kellogg said, "The orange is one of Nature's finest gifts to man." He had plenty of evidence to base this statement on as the juice of this fruit contains a predigested food in a most delicious form, ready for immediate absorption and utilization. They require no digestion and the sweeter the orange the greater its food value.

Oranges are an excellent source of Vitamin C (ascorbic acid) which is a specific remedy for scurvy. This one quality alone saved the lives of thousands when it was learned that citrus juice prevented scurvy. Consequently, in the early 1700's the British parliament adopted a law prescribing citrus juice for the British Navy. From then on, the antiscorbutic quality of oranges was accepted. Back in 1940 Dr. Russell Wilder, chairman of the nutrition committee, National Research Council, Washington, D.C., gave a command that U.S. soldiers were to receive four times as much vitamin C as previously given or the equivalent of an 8 ounce glass of fresh orange juice. This quantity was to prevent ills and to speed the healing of wounds.   *Dr. I. H. Nedge.*

Natural bioflavinoids are best obtained by eating much of the inner white portions of the rind. See under Grapefruit and Lemon.

OREGANO

The strongly aromatic Oregano has been found valuable as a stimulating carminative most useful in indigestion, dyspepsia, nausea and colic. For over 150 years it has been recognized for its pain-relieving action, which therapeutically is due principally to the content of the camphor found in the volatile oils. The oil is an active ingredient of proprietary "germicides" and as a pain-reliever of various liniments; for internal purposes, its carminative and diaphoretic properties are especially beneficial in indigestion, neuralgia and rheumatic conditions.

For comparative effects, a warm tisane of the herb is prepared by steeping half a teaspoonful in a cup of hot water, covered 5 minutes, stirred and steamed and *sipped slowly* every 2 hours or so. Not only has this tea been found beneficial for the relief of painful neuralgia, a poultice of the herbs may be applied as warm as possible to the face for several minutes every hour or as often as required. A heaping tablespoon of dried ground herbs is *moistened* with hot water, covered 10 minutes and more hot water added. Apply the mixture. The freshly made poultice is most beneficial for the quick relief of painful sprains, bruises, swellings, felon, etc.

"It is an excellent medicine in nervous cases. The leaves and tops dried and given in powder, are good in headaches of that kind. The tops made into a conserve are good for disorders of the stomach and bowels, such as flatulence and indigestion, and an infusion of the whole plant is serviceable in obstructions of the viscera, and against jaundice."

PAPAYA

Papain is the name generally given to the dried juice of the Papaya fruit *(Carica Papaya)* and in powdered form has been used in dyspepsia and gastric catarrh. It is claimed that "from time immemorial the fresh leaves of the Papaya plant have been used by the Indians to wrap meat in and to make it tender, and as a dressing to foul wounds."

Papaya—The Wonder Fruit. The papaya is one of our most important fruits, possessing extraordinary nutritive qualities. Richer in vitamins than almost any other fruit known, Papaya is noted for its abundance of A, C, and E vitamins, with calcium, phosphorus and iron as the leading minerals. Few edible foods contain so fine an assortment as this Wonder Fruit.

An interesting fact about the papaya is the lack of any noticeable amount of starch, either in the green or ripe fruit. Tests on many samples of ripe pulp have shown that starch was entirely absent. As to the sugar content, it is practically all of reduced sugars—simple forms which can be immediately absorbed by the blood, most of its elements have been already predigested by nature and its active enzyme principle aids the digestion of other foods entering the stomach with it.

In severe cases of digestive disorders, Papaya is invaluable because it can be retained in the stomach when other foods cannot be digested. The Bureau of Plant Industry, U.S. Department of Agriculture, states, "Papaya contains peculiar and valuable digestive properties which make it of great value in the diet; the fresh fruit is generally recognized as of value in promoting health."

There are numerous ways in which Papayas or their juice can be used in the daily dietary. They can be cut lengthwise and eaten with a spoon after the seeds and other unedible parts have been removed, or the entire fruit can be liquefied and wholly consumed.

Vegetarian News Digest.

The juice of this luscious fruit helps to correct intestinal disorders within a short time and taken upon an empty stomach has a pronounced tonic and rebuilding effect upon the entire digestive system. Powdered Papaya, actually the dried juice of the leaves and fruit, is used as a tenderizer of tough meats, and down South, chickens and pigs are fed the leaves to render their flesh more tender. And in Florida where I visited in 1959, I was told that the Seminole Indians apply the fresh leaf as a dressing to ulcers or open wounds.

The fresh fruit contains these valuables: Protein, citric, malic and tartaric acids, sodium, potassium, and phosphoric acid.

Here's How Papaya Helps

Gives quick relief in gastritis, dyspepsia and indigestion. Attacks and destroys dead tissue and false membrane in the digestive tract. Cleanses the intestinal tract of accumulated decayed and diseased matter. Aids normal body functions. Assures regularity of elimination. Acts as a healing agent to live tissues. Serves as an antidote against bowel and stomach disorders. Prepares food for ready assimilation. Furnishes many enzymes not found in most fruits. Supplies nearly every vitamin necessary for body nourishment. (A, C, E and D and K plus minerals such as calcium, iron and phosphorus.) Cuts excessive mucus. Assures an acid-alkaline balance. Forms amino acids by its action on protein. Guards against halitosis and offensive body odors. Cleanses the mouth and teeth. Aids in digesting foods for which there may be individual idiosyncrasies, such as milk, onions, garlic, cheese, etc. The unquestioned effectiveness of the Papaya as an antidote against many disorders of the digestive and intestinal tracts is attested to by those who through consistent use have proven this fact to their own satisfaction.   *Let's Live.*

PAPRIKA

See under Red Pepper.

"Go" for Green or Yellow: Natural color of a vegetable is an indicator of its vitamin A value. *The deeper the green or the yellow* of a vegetable, the more carotene (pro-vitamin A) it contains. This substance is called pro-vitamin A because from it the body can manufacture vitamin A. The more the intense color runs through the entire edible portion of the vegetable, the greater the nutritive value. This information came from *Nutrition Committee News U.S. Department of Agriculture,* Sept.-Oct. 1956.

PARSLEY

This is the common Parsley which is so extensively used as

a food and culinary herb. It has been in cultivation since early times and was held in high esteem by the ancient Greeks and Romans who included it as a part of their festive garlands because it retained its color so long. "Sweet and grateful to the stomach is Parsley," saith Galen nearly 1800 years ago. It is certainly a most health-fortifying food for all interested in fortifying their health and should be ever cultivated in one's garden, and yes, even in flower pots.

The leaves are indeed remarkable for their richness in carotene (Vitamin A) and ascorbic acid (Vitamin C), and an appreciable quantity of Vitamin B factors. Parsley contains these four vital minerals, calcium, copper, iron and manganese, the better to strengthen and "purify" your blood stream. Think twice before wasting Parsley as a garnish ("and who eats that ornament—that decoration?") or as a seasoning for soup or not eating it at all. It is one of the richest food sources of quickly absorbed vitamins and minerals, and offers at least 40,000 units of Vitamin A, more than 7 times that of Carrots and about 4 times that of Spinach.

Always eat Parsley uncooked—not as a culinary and not as a wasted garnish; and don't spoil its superb food value by including it in soups. And when you're having a lot of "raw" Onion or Garlic, do eat a handful of Parsley leaves to mask their tale-telling aroma.

Since earliest of days the leaves, seeds and roots of this all-purpose vegetable have been used for a variety of medicinal purposes: The aromatic "seeds" (actually fruits) were formerly considered useful to "disperse wind at the stomache and relieve those who are troubled with the cholic." But the seeds are better known as the commercial source of a substance today greatly used in Europe in malarial disorders.

Herbalist Culpepper had written that Parsley is very "comfortable to the stomach, good for wind and to remove obstructions both of the liver and spleen. The leaves laid to the eyes that are inflamed with heat or swollen, relieves them if it be used with bread. The seed is effectual to break the (kidney) stone and ease the pain and torments thereof. . . ."

However, the therapeutics of the roots, as described by Meyrick, are more to the point: "A strong decoction of the roots is a powerful diuretic, and is excellent in obstructions of the viscera, and such disorders as arise therefrom. Drank for some time, it is serviceable in the jaundice and dropsy, and brings away gravel and other fabulous concretions from the kidnies and bladder."

Today, as in former days, a decoction of the roots of 2 year old plants is used as a diuretic in mild dropsy and as an effective antilithic to remove gravel and stone from the kidney apparatus. To prepare the decoction, boil a tablespoonful of the dried, cut roots in a quart of hot water for 15-20 minutes. When cool, stir, strain and take cupful doses 3-4 times a day.

However, the dried leaves (also of the second year old plants) are far more commonly used for the same purposes as the roots and should be either steeped or simmered but not boiled (decocted). The infusion is prepared by stirring well one heaping teaspoonful in a cup of hot water and covering until cold. Stir, strain and drink one such cupful 4 times a day. Or a heaping tablespoonful of the leaves may be simmered in a quart of hot water for 30 minutes, covered until cool and strained. It is interesting to note that during the first World War, many English soldiers who fell victim to certain kidney disorders associated with dysentery, partook much of the aforementioned Parsley teas.

❧   ❧   ❧

PARSNIP

When carefully analyzed, these roots, which were highly esteemed and vastly cultivated by the Ancients, will be found to be highly concentrated in their food values far exceeding those of mostly all of our common vegetables except the Potato. An observation made by Herbalist Gerard is worth a quote: "The Parsnips nourish more than do the Turnips or the Carrots, and the nourishment is somewhat thicker, but not faultie nor bad. . . . There is a good and pleasant food or bread made of the roots of Parsnips. . . ."

Parsnips should be cooked quickly in a little boiling water for no longer than 8-10 minutes or baked until soft. They are best eaten with other vegetables and fat-less or non-flesh proteins. Although this food is low in sodium and calcium, it offers a very high content of chlorine, iron, magnesium, phosphorus, and potassium and especially sulfur and silicon. Because of the latter two elements, Parsnip juice, says Dr. R. D. Pope, is most valuable in correcting the condition of brittle nails and mild nervous disorders.

The fruits ("seeds") were formerly employed by herbalist and physician alike as a decoction to provide a gently stimulating diuretic which greatly helped to remove obstructions of the viscera. Dr. William Withering believed that the seeds contain an essential oil and will cure intermittent fevers or "agues"; and according to Dr. Meyrick, "a strong decoction of the root is a pretty strong diuretic, and assists in removing obstructions. . . . It is good against the jaundice and gravel."

It has been reported to me that a diet of Parsnips, steamed or baked, persistently and faithfully adhered to for lunch and dinner of 5 or 6 days, furnishes a highly prized diuretic, gentle and effective, to help better eliminate stone and accumulated toxins from the kidney apparatus.

❧　❧　❧

PEACH

Although all parts of the tree, leaves, kernels, flowers and bark, are therapeutically active, the first two generally furnish the parts used, for in them there is found the greater concentration of the active constituent, hydrocyanic acid. This is found also in two native herbal plants, Wild Cherry and Elder, the former having extensively served as an excellent sedative remedy for bronchitis, whooping and the usual cough, and the latter for colds, coughs and especially high blood pressure.

An infusion of the leaves, Dr. Brown stated, is a welcome remedy for bladder irritability and inflammation of the stomach and abdomen, and further lends its sedative, diuretic and slightly laxative qualities. A more recent writer claims that the syruped infusion furnishes one with demulcent, sedative, and expectorant qualities which help to greatly correct the irritation or congestion of the gastric membranes. To prepare the infusion, steep a tablespoonful of the leaves in a pint of hot water and cover until cold. Stir, strain and sip slowly a tablespoonful every hour as required. Up to a few years ago, a common household remedy for an ear-ache was a strong decoction of the leaves, and a few drops of the concentrated juice were dropped into the ear to effectively ease the pain.

As for the kernels, at the turn of the century they were often prepared into a tincture (alcoholic solution) or syrup and administered as a highly prized tonic in intermittent fevers. One commentator of these days advised his readers to put the kernels to further use by bruising or pounding them, then gently boiling in vinegar "to a thick paste or ointment which will cause the hair to grow upon bald places or where the hair is too thin." A variation of this recipe appeared recently in the *Boston Globe:* "To make hair grow put a measured gill of ripe peach meats and one pint of good vinegar into a bottle. Wash the spots where the hair has fallen off with this mixture three times a day, and the hair will soon grow."

(Do you remember how, during World War I, you performed one of your patriotic duties by saving all your Peach Kernels?)

When Peaches are in season—and theirs unfortunately is too short—be sure to eat much of these luscious fruits, which are best combined with Apples and Apricots and the native fruits of Blackberry and Raspberry, Mulberry, Elder and Huckleberry.

Peaches and blue Grapes bring iron to the blood. This iron, organized in vegetable cells, is therefore quickly assimilated. A whole meal of ripe Peaches in season will do good that lasts for a long time. People who eat great quantities of Peaches while they are to be had fresh, bring advantages to the body that will endure for a whole year.

❦   ❦   ❦

BLACK PEPPER

Kerdvic Frunz, Ph. T., of Springfield, Illinois, has suggested that to obtain relief of pain in the home treatment of rheumatism, neuritis, sprains, etc., one should use poultices of black Pepper, although any of the other strong spices may be similarly employed. Poultice-maker Frunz recommends this local application and says:

"For the treatment of pleurisy. It relieves the pain and congestion of pleurisy quickly as a rule, although internal treatment is usually indicated as well. Directions for the preparing of black Pepper poultice are given as follows: Place about a cup and a half full of ordinary cider vinegar in a basin and just bring it to a boiling point on the stove. When the vinegar comes to a boil simply sift in enough common black pepper to make a fairly thick paste, stirring well as the black pepper is added. This completed, spread the black pepper paste thus prepared on a piece of linen cloth just the right size to thoroughly cover the painful area, and then place the paste next to the skin, directly over the seat of the pain. Allow this to remain on for about three hours at the end of which remove by simply lifting up the corner of the cloth and then pull off quickly. Remove the surplus pepper remaining on the skin by washing with witch hazel. Never use water, as that would spoil the curative effects of the poultice."

Cataplasm of Black Pepper: This preparation is generally applied to the pit of the stomach in colic and cold, and may be used as a reliable replacement for the store-bought plaster.

Powdered Mustard	—4 ounces
Powdered Ginger	—1 teaspoonful
Black Pepper	—1 teaspoonful

Mix the spices and add enough warm water to produce a soft paste.

To prepare an ointment for ringworm of the scalp *(tinea capitis)*, incorporate 2 level teaspoonsful of the powdered spice into an ounce of lard, chicken fat or other non-petroleum (i. e. non-vaseline) base. Apply a small amount thoroughly into the scalp twice a day, morning and night.

PLEASE: To avoid possible gastric disturbances, season your foods *not* with Peppers—White, Black or Red, but with the delightfully flavorful and gentle aromatics, Basil, Marjoram, Thyme, Savory, et al.

While there are many remedies containing the Peppers intended for internal purposes, I cannot recommend them, for within these pages are many other remedies containing the gentle and equally efficacious herbal medications.

❧   ❧   ❧

RED PEPPER

Of all the members of the Capsicum family which claims the hot, Cayenne and the sweet California varieties of Red Pepper, Tabasco, Paprika and Pimiento (black and white Pepper belong to another family), only the California and the Pimiento varieties may be included in one's diet. They must not, however, be eaten at all when the digestive apparatus is upset or impaired to the slightest degree; and furthermore, the red, Cayenne variety must be eliminated from the menu, either as a food or condiment, that irritation to the gastric mucous membranes may be prevented. The fresh California may be cut lengthwise and included in the vegetable plate, and the Pimiento may be baked and served with either other warmed or salad vegetables.

Paprika or Hungarian Pepper, is decorative, a coloring aid and seasoning for meat and fish dishes and as such should be used *sparingly*. The powder is often used by bird fanciers to deepen the color of canaries.

The dried Red Pepper, whole or powder, provides the medicinal remedies which are intended mainly for external purposes. Not only is the powder included in bird foods, it also provides the chief ingredients of a warming powder which I have prepared for ice skaters for many years. Alone or diluted with an inert powder, it helps to warm chilled feet. Sprinkle a little in the shoes.

Red Pepper Cataplasm is prepared by mixing together 1 ounce of the powder, 3 ounces each of Mustard and Soap in 10 ounces of alcohol. This is an active rubefacient type of liniment.

Red Pepper Liniment: Warm 4 ounces each of turpentine and vinegar and add 1 tablespoonful of ground Pepper. When cool, add 4 ounces of rubbing grain alcohol and shake well. Cover and allow to ripen for 3 days, shaking occasionally. Strain and preserve in a well stoppered bottle.

That there is nothing new or original in medications, even in toothache remedies, is evidenced by Dr. Meyrick's direction for preparing such a poultice: "A little of the pulpy part of the fruit, held in the mouth, cures the toothache." The harshness of the spice, of course, will be lessened by the addition of the few dried bread crumbs or ground Sassafras, the herb which, I tell my students, should be called "the herb of a dozen uses." But it is far more interesting to note that the druggist today sells a dental poultice called Poloris which is much used for the relief of toothaches. This product contains principally Red Pepper, Sassafras and Hops.

That Pepper is used for various external purposes is further noted by Meyrick who advises its use as an application for quinsy throat: "Applied to the part affected in the form of a poultice, with the addition of crumbled bread, and honey enough to bring it to a proper consistence, it is good for the quinsy." Not only will the spice be found as the chief rubifacient in many proprietary rubs, Red Pepper Rub, Capsolin, and Methyl Rub, etc., internally, for sore or quinsy throat, the powder is often included in lozenges such as Throat Discs, manufactured by the Parke-Davis Co. that are intended to relieve the scratching and irritation of cough, sore throat, etc. I do not recommend the inclusion of such a harsh spice in any remedy for internal use.

A powder consisting of equal parts of borax and powdered Pepper becomes an excellent insect or ant deterrent. Slowly mix the two and spread lightly over the threshold.

PERSIMMON

When the fruits are green, they are quite astringent but when fully mature, and after being conditioned by the frost, they are most sweet and palatable. The globular fruits are dark yellow to orange when ripe, and being alkaline are eaten with the foods indicated under Peach.

In the Southeastern States the dried seeds are roasted and ground and used as a substitute for Coffee. The unripe green fruits, because of their high percentage of tannic and malic acids are used as an astringent in the usual bowel complaints, diarrhea, dysentery, etc. They may be used in an infusion of hot water or wine—3 fruits, cut in small pieces, to a cup of liquid. In using a wine base, allow the maceration for at least a day. The dose of either is a tablespoonful 3 or 4 times a day. . . . However, we have always considered a strong infusion an effective gargle for an ulcerated or sore throat.

PETROLATUM JELLY

See under Ointment Bases.

Proverb: Money is the most envied but the least enjoyed; health is the most enjoyed, but the least envied.

PINEAPPLE

The use of pineapple juice as an anthelmintic in Brazil and India, reports the *Journal of the American Pharmaceutical Association,* is supported by evidence that pineapple juice digests intestinal parasites in vitro. Canned juice does not have the same effect.

Mrs. Marion Tighe has written me: "The fresh juice of Pineapple has been proven for me a most effective remedy for sore and raspy throats when other remedies have not helped. It must, however, be fresh Pineapple. Canned or otherwise treated, it is of no use at all."

POMEGRANATE

"Eat the Pomegranate for it purges the system of hatred and envy." *Mohammed.*

The Bible tells us that King Solomon cultivated in his garden not only many of our everyday fruits and herbs, but an orchard of Pomegranate bushes. And Dr. Esser states that "when the children wandering in the Wilderness, sighed for the fleshpots of Egypt, it is certain that they much more longingly yearned for the refreshing Pomegranates, along with Figs, and Grapes."

In the countries to which it is indigenous, the fruit is eaten as a dessert and its juice is added to Summer beverages.

As for its medicinal benefits, its employment in the treatment of tapeworm was known to the ancients long before the learned physicians of Greece and Rome used this food as a worm-expellant. And although the root bark of the fruit has been used for centuries as an anthelmintic, i.e. tapeworm expeller, the rinds may be likewise employed. The fruit rinds are saved after eating the acidulous pulp, dried well and finely ground, and though their medicinal properties are somewhat less active than the roots, they may be substituted for the latter.

The anthelmintic properties are further commented upon by *The Dispensatory:* "The efficacy of its alkaloids, i.e. the active constituents, as taenicides has been abundantly confirmed and it appears to be established that the tannate of the alkaloids is the most effective and least dangerous form of the remedy—probably because its insolubility prevents its rapid absorption and enables it to come in prolonged contact with the worm."

Preparation: Two heaping teaspoonsful of the dried, finely ground rinds are slowly simmered for a half hour in two cups of hot water, contained in a porcelain or glass utensil. The patient having fasted at least half a day, or better still a full 24 hours, drinks two ounces of the cooled, strained liquid every hour for six doses beginning early morning. For better results, a brisk laxative should follow the last dose. This treatment continues the following two days, is stopped for three days, and again repeated for three mornings.

To prepare a gargle or canker remedy, boil 2 ounces or 2 tablespoonsful of the dried rind in 1½ pints of hot water down to one pint, strain and allow to cool. Use undiluted as a gargle for sore throat or as a wash or application to sore or bleeding gums. A member of our Herb Club suggests that the Rose Petals (dried) should be included in the above recipe, 2 heaping teaspoonsful to the original formula. Please note, that if this decoction is allowed to become more concentrated, the resultant liquid is an excellent remedy for simple diarrhea, suitable for young and old.

For summer fevers, there is nothing better than the juice of the Pomegranate to serve as a refrigerant, to lower the body temperature without the aid of chemical drugs, aspirin, etc. The many seeds are to be saved and dried and later incorporated into any demulcent-like remedy intended as an extra ingredient of a cough syrup, remover of catarrh from the mucous lining of the alimentary or urinary organs, etc.

🌷   🌷   🌷

POTATO

The potato ranks, as in my opinion, the most curative of all known food remedies. It may, indeed, seem a revolutionary idea that an exclusive potato regime can cure disease but such actually is the case. Such a diet has been found to possess remarkable powers of clearing away colds, fever, bronchial and digestive troubles, which for the most part, are due to an excess of acid poison waste in the system. Obstinate skin diseases of an intractible type and chronic nettle rash will yield to it when all other forms of treatment have failed.

The finest cleansing drink extant is that known as potato peel water. It is made from that part of the potato which contains the most nutriment but is usually discarded. A tumblerful of this beverage, made hot, should be taken during the day as the sole drink. An abundant flow of saliva, gastric and intestinal juices takes place. With these vital secretions also comes the pent up acid waste and toxins, the accumulation of which are the cause of the febrile or toxic condition of the body.

Dr. H. Valentine Knaggs.

Grated or shredded raw Potato, to further quote Dr. Knaggs, "makes an excellent fomentation to relieve rheumatic pains, bruises and some skin diseases."

Yes! Do eat this fine food steamed or baked. And *eat the skins,* for they offer high amounts of potassium, phosphorus, sulfur and chlorine.

No! Do not boil or fry the food since, if peeled and then boiled, it will lose 25-30% of potassium and at least 40% of the other elements. Fried foods are generally indigestible.

The juice of Potato, states one modern writer, is helpful

to those who suffer from gastric, nervous and muscular disturbances.

Warning: "The herbage (stems and leaves) appears at certain stages of growth to be toxic and severe cases of poisoning have been reported from (the eating of) Potato sprouts." And thus one must not partake of a Potato that shows the slightest color of green since then will it contain Solanine, a dangerous and poisonous alkaloid found in other members of the same nightshade family, such as Belladonna and Bittersweet.

Mrs. E. Pruneau, member of the Museum Herb Club, related her experience with the healing properties of friend Potato. The innocent victim by accidental scalding with hot water, she applied effective first aid to the severely burned forearm, a practice well remembered from early childhood. Her method was (and still is) to apply freshly cut thin slices of a large sized Potato to the affected area which in a day or so, was well on its healing way. And our members have likewise found that the mashed contents of an uncooked Potato also helps greatly to soothe recent burns and scalds.

Other of my notes refer to such home remedies as an arthritis poultice and an old fashioned remedy for erysipelas. To prepare the former, mix well an uncooked Onion and Potato, both finely ground; apply, keeping the mixture in place by means of cloth bandage. Every third application is alternated with a warm to hot poultice of Flaxseed. The erysipelas remedy is prepared by scraping a large sized Potato and applying it to the affected part. "Wrap it on carefully and keep on until the disease disappears."

Sometime ago I met a man who related a case of an old country woman who advised the eating of raw potatoes for the curing of eczema and other skin eruptions. He said that it worked miraculously in one case he knew of. I related this to one of the girls on our office force who had a severe case of eczema since a child. She was spending as much as $25.00 in one week for vitamin preparations which seemed to give her some relief. She discontinued the vitamins and after a few weeks on the raw potato diet, she obtained even better relief and she has been taking them ever since. It has not effected a complete cure but her face shows a remarkable change. She eats one raw potato a day.

Organic Gardening.

Heavily tarnished silver may be cleaned by soaking for two hours in potato water. Any remaining tarnish can be removed with a soft brush and silver polish.

❦   ❦   ❦

PRUNES

Before one eats Prunes, which are actually dried Plums (*Prunus Domestica*), they must be soaked in cold water for several hours, as must Raisins, which are dehydrated Grapes, Apricots and other commercially dried fruits. The water in which the fruit soaks the first hour is discarded, and thus is also discarded the greater portion of the sulphur dioxide, a chemical preservative with which the fruits are generally sprayed.

This food should be combined with Figs, Bananas, Apples, other Plums, Peaches and Grapes, and must be thoroughly masticated.

In their fresh and unfired state, Prunes contain a small amount of oxalic acid which in its natural state is of some benefit to the body, but it is little known that this same oxalic acid becomes a danger to the blood stream when the food (also Spinach, Rhubarb, et al) in which it appears, is boiled. The free acid then becomes very destructive to the blood's calcium supply. Therefore, do eat the fruit uncooked, uncomposted and untampered with.

Prunes have long been regarded as a laxative remedy and were an ingredient of Confection of Senna which until a few years ago, enjoyed widespread popularity among the medical practitioners and lay folks. The confection has made an interesting come-back in recent years because of its herbal ingredients: Senna, Coriander, Figs, Tamarind, Cassia, Prunes and Licorice.

❦   ❦   ❦

PUMPKIN SEEDS

The ripe seeds of this late summer garden product have been used successfully for many years as a worm expellant or in combination with Pomegranate fruit rind and Male Fern root. There are two ways of administering the seeds as medicine, by chewing the shelled seeds or by preparing a syrup of them. The former method is preferable. The dose is one or two ounces shelled and chewed well, every hour for three hours; skip three hours and resume the dose again every hour for three doses, doing this every other three hours for three days. Skip three days and resume the treatment. Remember that the seed embryo and green membrane must be well chewed.

To prepare a syrup, shell and bruise two ounces of the ripe seeds. They should be finely ground in a mortar or put through a meat grinder. Stir with a thick syrup of brown sugar or honey and flavor with powdered Cinnamon.

Yes, Squash seeds may be substituted for Pumpkin.

Worm Syrup Formula of the Laxol Company, New Haven, Conn.: Pumpkin Seed, Senna, Worm Seed, Sodium Bicarbonate, Peppermint, Anise Seed, Rochelle Salt, Sugar, Wintergreen.

"Now comes evidence from Germany showing that Pumpkin seed is beneficial in keeping the prostate gland in good shape," reports *Prevention.*

Prepare Pumpkin by steaming it only long enough to soften this food. Don't make a mish-mush of it.

❧   ❧   ❧

QUINCE

"Quinces not only yield pleasure but Health."

Neighbor John had cultivated the Quince, merely as an ornamental shrub and since had made no use whatsoever of the handsome fruits, not even as organic fertilizer, he most generously permitted me to gather as much of the ripening fruits as I desired. Nor could I resist offering a bit of pro-herb propaganda, for I assured him that a five minute demonstration to his three women folk would certainly have them appreciate the cornucopia of values that are offered by this valuable and desirable shrub.

It is admitted, though, that the Quinces that are cultivated here in New England yield such fruits which, when ripe, are somewhat tough, acidulous and I further confess, to some degree, unpalatable. However, after tasting a sample of our home-made Quince preserve and using our Komar

Hand Lotion, friend John now guards his Quince shrubs *and each fruit* most zealously.

How true are Herbalist Parkinson's words that "there is no fruit grown in the land that is of so many excellent uses as this, serving as well to make many dishes for the table, as for banquets and much for their physical virtues." Quinces yield a deliciously tart jelly and marmalade, prepared via the conventional recipes, either alone or with Apples, Lemons or Oranges. The fruits contain a substantial amount of protein, mucilage and malic acid. It is interesting to note that the English word marmalade is derived from the Portuguese, Marmelo, a Quince, and actually should be classified as the conserve (syrup)of Quince.

It is the inodorous seeds that are much more utilized as remedies. They resemble those of the Apple, and being highly mucilaginous, possess demulcent and soothing properties. We have prepared a soothing hand lotion by boiling a few seeds and 2 inch-size flakes of Tragacanth (or a teaspoonful of Irish Moss) in hot water, straining when cold, and thinning out the solution with a little glycerin. And a thick Quince base, syruped with brown sugar or Honey has proven its worth as a most acceptable demulcent drink to be taken during a convalescent period following feverish colds or temporary stomach disorders. For this purpose, use two teaspoonsful to a pint of hot water. This syrup is also well suited as a suspending agent for Tincture of Benzoin Compound (which see), which is often prescribed by physicians for laryngitis and hoarseness of the throat. Use ½ teaspoonful of the Tincture to 4 ounces of syrup. Sip it slowly.

Thin Mucilage of Quince Seeds: Mix well a heaping teaspoonful of the seeds in half cup of hot water, cover until cool and strain. This remedy, states Dr. Meyrick, "is an excellent medicine for sore mouths" and may be used with advantage to soften and moisten the (sore) mouth and throat infections. This makes a good wave-set for milady.

Mucilage of Quince Seeds: Digest one ounce of seeds (by weight) in a glass of boiling water for an hour. Strain. Not only is this preparation useful as an eye drop to remove foreign matter, it should be used as a base for cough syrups. Mixed with an equal part of Honey, it is used in hourly teaspoonful doses to relieve a cough or hoarseness. Store in refrigerator.

Bandoline for Hair: Mix equal parts of mucilage of Quince Seeds and Cologne Water (or perfumed Bay Rum diluted with an equal amount of water.) Use this as an application for the hair, to give it smoothness and gloss. Note: Do not confuse Quince with Quinsy Berries which are Black Currants.

Better be fit than fat; the fat man is the doctor's best friend.

RADISH

It is a little known fact that for centuries the pungent roots of this annual have been used as a source of medicine. To quote briefly from Meyrick's remarks, we find that "the juice of radish root, newly expressed with the addition of a little wine, is a notable remedy for the gravel, scarce anything operates more speedily by urine or brings away fabulous concretions more effectually. The roots eaten plentifully sweeten the blood and juices, and are good against the scurvy."

According to *The United States Dispensatory*, the juice of the well known plant has been used by Grumme in the treatment of cholelithiasis, a condition in which concretions are present in the gall-bladder or bile ducts. As an aid in preventing the formation of biliary calculi, (gallstones) he employed the expressed juice of the crushed roots in doses of 2 to 4 ounces.

And, too, we learn that the Radish was rather popular as a food and medicine in early Rome and Greece and was highly recommended by the physicians of both lands as an eye opener, to be eaten uncooked with bread in the early Summer.

Grow your own Radish roots. Collect them for the table when they're young or else they will contain far too much of the woody fibers which are often difficult to digest. Please remember that *if the roots are too pungent to the taste, it is better to leave them alone.*

The top greens (of your own garden grown crop) should not be discarded as worthless for they are an excellent source of food. For table use, they should be steamed 3-4 minutes in the water with which they are washed. Season with Lemon juice or herb vinegar. Son Saul now agrees that "well, *that way,* they don't taste bad at all."

Try the very young greens *uncooked,* mixed into a salad.

❦ ❦ ❦

RASPBERRY

The fruits are often used in the preparation of home-made jams and jellies but should be eaten uncooked whenever possible, if one is to benefit from all of the nutritive values of this ubiquitous native. An excess may be included in the manufacture of an herb wine, or else dehydrated and saved for future use. The dried leaves serve well as a tea substitute, when mixed with Mint, dried Lemon or Orange peels.

Raspberry fruits contain fruit sugar, pectin, proteins, citric and malic acids, a high percentage of Vitamin C and minerals, magnesium, calcium, phophorus, sodium, chlorine, potassium and sulfur. They are therefore alkaline in reaction, cooling and fragrant and should be eaten with other sub-acid fruits as Apples, Grapes or Plums.

Medicinally, the freshly expressed juice has been extensively employed by European doctors in the treatment of scrofula. The juice has been also used since Elizabethan days as a specific remedy to dissolve the tartar of the teeth. For that purpose, eat much of the raw fruits when in season.

In feverish colds, a heaping tablespoon of the fresh fruits may be boiled in 2 glasses of hot water for 10 minutes, strained and allowed to cool. The dose is a half cupful every hour. A stronger decoction is useful in simple diarrhea.

The name Fragrarine, reports *Drug Topics,* has been given by Sir Beckwith Whitehouse to the active principle of Raspberry leaf extract, which is being used, experimentally in this country, in allaying the pains of labor. The extract appears to relax the uterine muscles.

❦ ❦ ❦

RHUBARB

True, this plant is rich in much-needed elements of minerals and vitamins but since its oxalic acid content is far too excessive, it must be considered as an undesirable source of nutrient, when prepared via the usual boiling-spoiling way.

RICE

Unrefined brown Rice is well known for its nutritive components especially the members of the vitamin B family. An emollient decoction of the grains has long been taken as nutriment by the convalescent, when other foods could not be tolerated. For this purpose, Rice water or gruel is generally prepared, but often the mixture is allowed to be reduced to a "pap" which on cooling, becomes a moderately consistent jelly. The resultant jelly is a source of good diet in dyspepsia and intestinal complaints.

Rice Diet Successful in Treating Disease

A new report on the successful use of a diet of rice to treat heart and kidney disease was made not long ago at the annual meeting of the American College of Physicians. The rice diet, according to Dr. Walter Kempner, Associate Professor of Medicine, Duke University, is based on the theory that *salt, protein and fat are detrimental in large quantities and their restriction is warranted in the treatment of disease of the blood vessels, resulting from high blood pressure and hardening of the arteries.* (My italics)

Dr. Kempner said that the diet is very low in salt and protein and cholesterol, a fatty substance which experimentally has been found to produce hardening of the arteries. He said that a study of almost 1,000 patients showed that the rice diet acts beneficially to reduce the blood cholesterol in a great majority of patients and in many to a significant degree.

The greatest number of successful results came in from those who followed the diet the longest. (My italics). He said "the rice diet also has brought benefits in chronic nephritis, or Bright's disease, and in edema or dropsy." *Vegetarian News Digest.*

The Rice diet can hardly be considered revolutionary for hypertension or high blood pressure sufferers. Rice is no "miracle food" and should not be expected to be a "cure" or even a treatment in the lowering of blood pressure. Dr. Kempner's rice diet included "a cupful of unsalted rice (dry weight) per day or ⅓ pound at each meal and as much fresh fruit and juice as desired, a handful of sugar and vitamin in tablet form." Do substitute Honey, or Molasses for white sugar which although considered an important (?) source of energy in the rice diet, may eventually obviate the entire regimen. For synthetic vitamin pills, do substitute fresh organically grown fruits and vegetables.

Rough, Whole Grain Brown Rice—One of Most Nutritive Foods

The unpolished whole grain brown rice is the real rice and is one of our finest foods. . . . Demineralizing the food means demineralizing the blood and organs and thus making them more susceptible to disease.

The amount of mineral matter found in a thousand parts of water-free whole rice as compared with other foods shows that the rice contains more potassium than corn meal or barley, twice as much potassium as cow's butter and a seventh more phosphorus than potatoes. Compared with polished rice it has four times as much potassium, four times as much magnesium, four and a half times the amount of iron, phosphorus, and calcium, more than three times as much sulphur, sodium, and silicon and twice as much chlorine.

Unpolished brown rice also contains the fat soluble vitamin A which is the growth promoting vitamin. The lack of the A vitamin will in time produce a disease of the eyes. The evidence of this disease which is caused by malnutrition is shown by granular lids and sore eyes. Unpolished brown rice also contains water soluble vitamin B known as the anti-neuritic vitamin which has an important bearing on health. The lack of this vitamin tends to bring on gastro-intestinal troubles, neuritis, loss of weight, anemia, and the general breaking down of the organic functions of the body.

Brown unpolished rice is especially good as a food in cases of irritation of tissues of the mouth, aesophagus, and stomach and also for kidney disorders. Rice is like milk (Ed. whole) in that its decomposition products have no real injurious effects upon the kidneys, and they may be eaten together by people suffering from nephritis without harmful effects. People with poor digestion will also find that properly prepared rice is easily digested and forms a highly desirable food. All kinds of stomach and intestinal disorders may be benefitted by eating Brown unpolished rice. Since it does not form uric acid, its use should be encouraged in cases of gout; it is also an excellent food for those suffering from heart trouble, blood vessel complaints and liver ailments.

From *Brown Rice Research.*

Neuritis: Question: What foods are good for recurring attacks of neuritis? Is there any proof that such foods as rice polishings are good for a condition like that? Miss F. A.

Answer: As far back as 1911 Funk discovered that he could paralyze pigeons by neuritis by feeding them on polished rice. Then he could make it possible for them to walk and fly within a few hours by giving a substance made from rice bran and yeast. He called this organic substance by the new name of vitamine. His theory was that the lack of vitamine in the food makes it necessary for the body to get the substance from its own tissues and this results in a wasting of the muscles and a breaking down of nerve tissues in those muscles. *Maydene Williamson.*

❦ ❦ ❦

ROSE

The hay-feverite may prepare a home remedy for sore and irritated eyes by steeping a few Rose petals in a cup of hot water. A drop or two of the carefully filtered liquid will then be applied to each eye 4 or 5 times a day. One of the most widely used proprietary remedies employed as an eye drop for the relief of hay fever is the druggist's Estivin which is a "processed infusion of Rose petals" manufactured by the Schieffelin Company. "In moderate cases of hay fever, a single drop of Estivin applied to the inner corner of each eye 3 times a day is sufficient to control eye and nose symptoms and to keep the patient comfortable."

The dried petals and leaves are often used with Peppermint, Lemon Peel, and Linden leaves as a tea substitute, especially adapted for folks with arthritis or dyspepsia, and for others who cannot tolerate the excessive tannic acid of tea or coffee or who do not wish to ingest the heart-stimulating caffeine of those beverages. Rose petals contain malic and tartaric acids, said to be of great value in dissolving out gallstones and gravel from the urinary organs.

However, the hips, as the fruits are commonly called, have recently come into prominence as a superior, natural source of Vitamin C, possessing 60 times as much as Lemons possess. Appreciable quantities of citric and malic acids and natural sugar are also present. Each fruit is reported to yield 10 mg. of Vitamin C. And British scientists have also found that these fruits are good sources of Vitamins A and P. The latter is present in the peel of most citrus fruits, plays an important role in the prevention of rupture and bleeding of the minute capillary vessels, and aids the healing of wounds.

❦   ❦   ❦

ROSEMARY

> "Rosemarine is for remembrance
> Between as daie and night,
> Wishing that I may alwaie have
> Your present in my sight."
> *Sir Thomas More.*

The pungency of its aromatic oil must have been familiar to the Europeans of the past few centuries. There are many references to show that they were quite familiar with the disinfective and germicidal properties of the herb of which they made profitable use by strewing the freshly cut plant upon the floors of churches and meeting places, and on such occasions as weddings and funerals. Thus one discovers the reason for Rosemary's being employed by the superstitious Italian and Spaniard of the dark ages—"To ward off the evil spirits," by sprinkling the herb in places where they imagined the mal-doer lurked ready to spread disease and evil. Yet, until very recently a mixture of Rosemary and Juniper berries was the only preparation used in many of the French Hospitals to cleanse the sick-rooms of foul odors and prevent the spreading of contagious infections.

The French call it the Incensier Method, the same

method that was employed centuries ago: Take a handful each of Juniper fruits and crushed Rosemary herb and stir them well in a pan containing about a quart of hot water, which is kept over a radiator, or stove, during the winter. In the Summer herb sprigs may also be stationed in the direct path of the sun rays and before long, the bonodorous steaming herb vapors containing minute quantities of volatile oil of Rosemary and Juniper will extend their antiseptic benefits throughout the room and the air will be soon cleansed of stale, foul odor. In his *Theatricum Botanicum,* Mr. Culpepper tells that "to expell the contagion of the pestilence burne the hearbe in Houses and chambers in the time of infection to correct the aire in them."

The Incensier method is crude—old-fashioned? Perhaps so although you too, will find this method works out so satisfactorily that you will recommend this method to others. Better still, read the label of two popular germicide sprays sold in the drugstore, Dr. Hubbard's and Red Cross Germicides, and you will be reminded that the active ingredients are oils of Lavender, Pine, Cajeput, and friend Rosemary. Use the French Incensier method wherein fresh (preferable) herbs are utilized at very little cost or trouble and you may practically derive the same approximate results derived of the commercial alcoholic disinfectants aforementioned.

Yes, a present day herbal authority tells us:

Growing on sandy soil, it is rich in silicon salts, which in old age are said to drain from the body; their place often being filled with calcium salts. As one of the herbs of old age with failing memory and stiff joints, Rosemary brings added mobility and lively intellect. Grecians drank it to clear the head and to facilitate mental labor. An infusion delighteth the head and is wonderfully refreshing to tired business men and students. It is as natural an antidote to mental fatigue and it also strengthens sight. It is known to restore speech after a stroke. [See Tisane.] Arabians used to sprinkle the powdered herb on wounds and also used it as an insecticide.

Arnoldu de Villa Nova advised inhaling the fumes of ignited Rosemary or dried Cedarwood for influenza and for the speedy relief of colds. Burning Rosemary was used for many years as a prophylactic.

We are told by the herbalists of former days that "the distilled water of the flowers of Rosemary taketh the stench (of the mouth) away, i.e. this solution helps to overcome "halitosis," for which purpose herbs Anise and Mint are also indicated in the following recipe.

Mouth Wash: Steep ¼ to ⅓ teaspoonful of each herb in a cup of hot water, cover for 10 minutes and strain. Rinse the mouth and/or use as a gargle every hour retaining the solution as long as possible, and should a little be accidentally swallowed, only good can come of it. This wash is recommended also for bleeding gums and sore throat.

Tisane: Mix ⅓ to ½ teaspoonful of this and then balance with one or two of your tisane favorites, in a cup of hot water for 5 to 6 minutes. Then strain. Sip the tea in driblets. Prepared with Mint and Sage, the tea "helpeth cold disease of the head" (headache) and calms the nerves, thus its popularity as a specific remedy for nervous headaches, although it is not usually included in the category of "medicinal herbs."

It may also be mixed with ground leaves of Mullein and Coltsfoot and employed in cases of bronchitis or asthma.

Cough Syrup: Mix well ½ part of Rosemary with one part each of Mullein and Hoarhound (or Coltsfoot) and steep a teaspoonful of the mixed herbs in a cup of hot water. Allow to cool and strain through absorbent cotton. Add enough sugar or honey to make a syrup. The dose is a tablespoonful sipped slowly, 3 to 4 times a day as required.

Hair Tonic: To prepare a desirable after-shampoo rinse for all shades of hair, infuse one ounce of Sage and Rosemary in a pint of hot water for 24 hours, stirring the mixture occasionally. Strain and add one teaspoonful of powdered borax. This Solution may also be employed as a "hair tonic" for loose dandruff or itchy scalp. (See under Castor Oil.)

For those bald spots or tendency to baldness, this preparation may be used: Mix well 4-5 drops of Oil of Rosemary with ½ ounce each of Castor Oil and unsalted lard (or Goose fat). Massage the scalp vigorously, a little of the preparation being used 3 times a day.

Moth Preventative and Insect Chaser: Use equal parts

of Rosemary, Lavender and ground Lemon peel. The trio offers itself also as a sachet to milady.

Notes: Recently, many bee-keepers of California have taken to the cultivation of Rosemary so that its distinctive flavor may be imparted to the resultant honey. To ease the irritation caused by Nettle rash and by insect bites, rub in fresh leaves of the herb. Violin makers finish their products with a special varnish of amber and oils of Linseed, turpentine and Rosemary.

🌷 🌷 🌷

SAFFRON

"Thy plants are an orchard of Pomegranate with pleasant fruit: Camphire with Spikenard and Saffron, Calamus and Cinnamon, with all trees of Frankincense, Myrrh, and Aloe, with all the chief spices."

Song of Solomon, 4: 13-14.

The herb was well known not only to the ancient Hebrews as the *Karkom* of the *Song of Solomon* and to the Romans and the Greeks (Ktokes) as shown in the writings of Hippocrates, Theophrastus and Theocritus. The Arabic elements called it *Sahafaran* or *Zafran,* which is derived from *Asafar,* yellow. There are many notices in herbal literature of its economic uses in everyday practice long before Westward-Ho Columbus set sail for foreign spice-laden lands, for in the early 1400's the orange-colored stigmas were found to be best in dyeing silk yellow. Even then it was considered an expensive article of trade and was much sought after by the tradesmen of other nations. And in the early 1900's the feathers of various birds were dyed yellow with the herb which also "constituted the vegetable dye of Spanish Vermillion, employed by ladies to lighten their complexions."

Medical writers for centuries have heaped well-earned praise upon the herb for its therapeutic efficacy, to wit: John Gerard said, "For those at death's doore and almost past breathing, Saffron bringeth breath again." And Dr. William Meyrick, friend of Dr. Withering, "It is thorough (in action) and a useful aromatic." . . . "In moderate doses this

substance (the stigmas) stimulates the stomach, has a spec-
ifying influence on the cerebrospinal system and has a result
analogous to that produced by other odorous flowers."

"In a medicinal point of view it is frequently used to
assist the eruptions of exanthematous diseases." It has a
strong penetrating smell, a warm pungent bitterish taste and
promotes easy perspiration.

Present-day herbalists and herb-users are well aware of
the therapeutic thoroughness of the usable part of this welcome harbinger of Spring. It is an established fact that, as
in past centuries, the stigmas are today (and should be)
employed to excellent advantage as a non-irritating diaphoretic in scarlet fever and measles. For this purpose, steep a
teaspoonful of Catnip (and one of Yarrow if available)
and ⅛ teaspoonful of Saffron in a cup of hot water. Stir well
and cover 8-10 minutes; stir and strain. The dose is one
such cupful every hour for 3 doses, one every 2 hours for 3
doses, then one 3 or 4 times a day.

🌷   🌷   🌷

Sign on the wall in the office of the *Vegetarian News Digest:*
A THINKING DRIVER DOESN'T DRINK;
A DRINKING DRIVER DOESN'T THINK.

🌷   🌷   🌷

SAGE

Sage is a *must* for gardener and householder. John Evelyn
had well noted that " 'tis a plant, indeed, with so many and
wonderful properties that the assiduous use of it is said to
render man immortal."

It is customary for most kitcheneers to make use of the
herb only for the turkey dinners on Thanksgiving and Christ-
mas, but during the other 50 weeks of the year Sage is needlessly neglected when it should be more profitably employed,
as Mr. Evelyn has just said.

Behold Sage!—an herb that is fast becoming more and
more indispensable as a culinary and medicinal, offering for
use its superb disease-preventing, health-fortifying properties
to the human body. Its health-saving influence may well be

interpreted by these two proverbs: "How can a man die who has Sage in his garden?" (Arabian) and "He that would live for aye Must eat Sage in May." (Old English).

Thus, the herbalist will recommend that one should drink warm teas of Sage three or four times a day during the few weeks of Spring from March 15 to the third or fourth week of May, and during every month of the calendar. Steep a level teaspoonful in a cup of hot water 10 minutes. Keep the cup covered with a saucer. Stir and strain. Drink one such cupful as often as desired. This herb infusion (tisane) performs as a good old Spring tonic reliable, and will do wonders to tone up the system and get rid of that leftover winter lethargy, that one may live "for aye," or at least to a fairly ripe old age.

Sage herb provides a most desirable substitute for tea or coffee when the caffeine of the latter creates too excitant an effect, in cases of nervous disorders or general digestive weakness. For meal time drinks, use about ½ teaspoonful of Sage either alone or with equal portions of Mint and ground Lemon peel. A little hot vinegar added to this warm compound provides a good application for sprains, bruises, etc. Apply to the affected parts as a compress as warm as can be tolerated.

Also interesting to note: The Chinese prized quite highly and even preferred Sage to their own tea. This herb provided for them as it may for us, a gently stimulating tonic and a sense of well-being when sipped in the manner of a mealtime beverage—and it is recorded that in trading with the early Dutch traders, they were willing to accept one pound of Sage for three of their own Pekoe.

One of my radio listeners, a beginner in herb usage writes, "I tried something new for a warm drink, a tea of Sage leaves. I do recommend that the listeners of your program do try it. It is delicious. Sage tea recalls many an herb remedy of my childhood days."

Many are the profitable uses of this rather prodigious herb and much has been written of its many and valued medicinal actions during the centuries of its known existence. To my grandparents, Sage was a near cure-all, and entered into most formulae intended for internal purposes, yes—52 weeks of the year.

Gargle and Canker Wash: Ingredients: 1 oz. of Sage and Sumac Berries, and ½ oz. of Goldthread (optional). Boil Sumac and Goldthread in 1½ pints of hot water for a half hour, add Sage and simmer another ½ hr. Strain and use warm.

Attention, Boy Scouts:—This solution is equally effective as a dressing application to scratches or wounds.

Nervine (General Nerve Tonic): Catnip—4 parts, Sage— 2 parts, Valerian—2 parts, Skullcap—4 parts, Chamomile —4 parts. Add a heaping teaspoonful to a cup of hot water and cover half an hour. Stir, strain and drink a wineglassful every 2 or 3 hours, if the condition so warrants. Otherwise, drink a cupful four times a day.

General Stomachic (For Nervous Stomach or Dyspepsia): Sage—1 part (or teaspoonful), Catnip—2 parts, Mint—2 parts, Linden—2 parts. Teaspoonful of herbs to a cup of hot water and cover 20 minutes. Stir, strain and drink ½ cupful as necessary or ½ hour before and after meals.

Diaphoretic (Sweating Agent in Systemic Colds): Use equal parts of the above mentioned ingredients, (Stomachic) and of Boneset and Yarrow, add 2 parts of each and prepare as before. Cover for 10 minutes only and drink one full cupful every hour or oftener until desired effects result. This formula will provide more than an ounce of prevention against possible winter colds if taken morning and night. (See also under Cinnamon).

Hair Tonic (See under Castor Oil).

❦   ❦   ❦

SALT

Table Salt, Sodium Chloride, is a great irritant, a mineral poison, and contrary to the accepted belief, never serves as nourishment for any part of the body. A result of improper, and over-cooking of foods is the addition of salt and is generally though improperly considered proper, plus the ubiquitous exaggerations of already misleading advertising claims. Over-cooking and moreover, over-boiling of foods, results in the partial loss of all the important vital mineral elements and especially the vitamins D, A, and C which are quickly destroyed by heat. The loss also includes the Vitamin B group.

The dangers of using salt as seasoning for table use need be emphasized, if only that it is a dangerous chemical without which the human body can do very well. That salt, as the commercial product, "improves digestion" is open to serious debate. This chemical is not only unsuitable for the human body; it interferes with normal digestion of foods by decreasing by ⅓ to ½, the action of the enzyme pepsin which is needed to digest the protein intake.

The use of the chemical as a seasoner at meal time or for whatever culinary purpose, is a gastronomic sin and can lead only to disastrous organic ailments. Little wonder then, that millions of Americans are now and ever on a salt-free diet, they whose every meal had been at one time well dosed with this toxic chemical, they who suffer the torments and the aches and pains of their respective ailments, be it heart trouble, high blood pressure, obesity, nephritis, diabetes or arthritis. Thus, to prevent the possibility of internal disorders, one should consider salt, the chemical, as an undesirable source of seasoning and taste.

Dr. Henry Gilbert reminds us that salt helps cause constipation, eczema, kidney troubles, eye infections, hardening of the arteries, etc. He says that a cancer specialist at the National Biochemical Laboratory contends that salt also causes cancer.

"It is common knowledge that salt may cause constipation, eczema, kidney trouble, hardening arteries and eye infections. Dr. Percy Robinson, of the National Biochemical Laboratory, Mount Vernon, who specializes in cancer contends that it also may cause that dread disease."   *Dr. Henry Gilbert.*

It is further recommended that one avoid table salt either as a seasoner in the salt-shaker or via potato chips, salted nuts or crackers, pretzels, popcorn, or salted fish or meat.

No less an accepted authority than *The Dispensatory* notes that "while sodium chloride is not generally regarded as a poison, it will be noted that it is capable of causing serious and often fatal poisoning, not only through its local irritant action upon the alimentary tract when swallowed but also because of its systemic effects. When large quantities are swallowed, the symptoms are nausea, vomiting and sometimes purging. The treatment should be administration of large quantities of water."

Sodium chloride occurs as natural sodium and chlorine, in adequate amounts to more than satisfy one's daily salt requirements, in all fresh fruits and vegetables, egg whites, dairy products, sea foods, meats and molasses. At meal-time, we may all enjoy the organic salt occurring as sodium (and) chloride in Nature-all fresh, uncooked Spinach, Parsley and Celery and other greens.

How then season cooked foods? Says Chef Pierre, "The important fact for the kitcheneer to remember is that the additions of culinary herbs to warm dishes (foods prepared with heat) emphasize but do not disguise the original flavor of foods. How often, sad to say, is the reverse too true!"

Examples of culinary herbs: Sage, Marjoram, Anise, Basil. Do try them. Do use Basil, Thyme, Marjoram and Sage and you too, will wonder where these wonderful flavorings have been all your life.

Several commercial herb salts as Celery and Garlic salt, unfortunately, contain the undesirable chemical salt, sodium chloride, which must be eliminated from one's diet altogether and substituted with health fortifying herbs. Powdered Mono-Potassium Glutamate may also be used. It is a vegetable derivative and though it possesses no flavor, it does tend to accentuate the diminishing positive of cooked foods. Use powdered Kelp and other herb powders as your seasoners.

As a medicinal agent, Salt has several applications, but principally for external purposes:

1. As an antidote for several poisons accidentally swallowed. It is here used for its quick active emetic property. The dose: A tablespoon dissolved in a cup of warm water.

2. It is often employed as a warm fomentation to relieve congestion and exudation and is useful therapy also for newly acquired sprains and bruises.

3. A quickly prepared nose drop requires only the dissolving of a few grains of the fine salt in a teaspoonful of tap water. Four or five drops in each nostril helps to relieve the congestion of the nasal passages due to colds, hay fever, etc.

4. A tablespoonful each of Epsom and table salt dissolved in a cup of hot water serves well as a soak for felons and boils.

As a warm fomentation to sprains and painful bruises, the following formula may be used: Dissolve two ounces of salt in six of warm water and mix with an equal portion of Vinegar. Apply as wet compress, preferably with turkish towel.

6. Coarse, dry salt, heated in a pan, may also be used as an application to bruises, sprains, etc. However, it is best

applied when contained within heavy cloth material, stocking or a towel.

7. And one of the best applications of chemical salt is its use in winter time to dissolve the treacherous ice.

❦　❦　❦

"You cannot avoid death but you can, through sensible living, push that end away for many, many years."

Frederick W. Collins.

❦　❦　❦

SESAME OIL

By all means do use this oil as a more healthful substitute for Olive Oil.

❦　❦　❦

SOAP

This product is more than a mere household commodity; it serves indeed as a priceless source of many worthy household remedies. It has admirably benefitted the kitchen chemist as a jiffy remedy for poison ivy and as an ingredient in an ointment for the itch and boils. For the latter purpose it is later indicated under cataplasm of soap and is also to be used as a plaster. It is frequently employed to relieve constipation resulting from hardened feces in the rectum, and for this purpose a solution of white soap (a level teaspoonful of finely ground soap is dissolved in a pint of warm water) is used as an enema morning and night.

It must be remembered that until recently soap had long been recognized by the medical and pharmaceutical laity as an important ingredient of laxatives and purgatives, gall bladder, kidney and "alterative" preparations. In the past in pharmacy according to some authorities, soap was often used for the purpose of giving a proper consistency to pills (aloes). In formulas intended for external use it is an excellent emulsifying agent, and is therefore indicated in the various formulae of the *U. S. Pharmacopoeia* and the *National Formula* of the doctor and druggist. And in addition, because Oleic acid does not ionize, soap gives us a useful way in which to neutralize mineral acids and metallic salts, and it is also a useful antidote in cases of poisoning by these agents. Also since there is an absence of effervescence in this reaction, it is considered a better agent for this purpose than the carbonates. The manner of administration in these cases is to give a teacup of a strong solution of soap every 3 or 4 minutes, until the patient has taken as much as he can swallow.

Alkaline Tooth Powder: Precipitated Chalk (Calcium Carbonate), 7 parts; Pure Castile Soap, 1 part; Mix well. To provide flavor, add only enough of an aromatic oil as Wintergreen, or Spirits of Peppermint, Wintergreen or Anise.

Camphorated Soap Liniment: Soap—3 ounces, Camphor—1 ounce, Alcohol—16 ounces, Aromatic Oil—2 teaspoonsful, Rosemary or Wintergreen. Gently warm the alcohol and in it, dissolve the soap. When the solution is cool, add the Camphor and Oil and dissolve. This liniment has been and still is much used as a "gentle rubefacient embrocation in sprains, bruises and rheumatic or gouty pains. It is largely used as a vehicle for more active (stronger) counter-irritants."

Chloroform Liniments: Camphorated Soap Liniment—15 ounces, Chloroform—½ ounce. This remedy is generally employed for the relief of painful bruises, and minor forms of myalgias, neuralgias, etc.

Cataplasm (Plaster) of Soap: Brown Soap—½ ounce, Rosated (or steamed) Onion—2 ounces, Ground Mustard—2 ounces, Water—enough. 2 ounces of sugar may be also added to this formula.

Heat together and mix into a cataplasm. Use as a maturating application to boils, abscesses, etc.

Poison Ivy Antidote: This remedy offers quick relief for itching and dermatitis due to the trio of public nuisances, Poison Ivy, Poison Sumac and Poison Oak. It is important to apply hot soap solution within one or two days after the rash has appeared.

Use Brown Soap, Fels Naphtha or Kirkman's. Place several thin strips, about ¼ of the bar, in a pint of hot water contained in a porcelain or pyrex pot, stir well and allow the soap to remain undisturbed for 3 or 4 minutes. Then agitate the mixture with a spoon until the soap is entirely dissolved. Apply the solution as hot as possible to the affected area. Do this 4-5 times a day.

Our favorite herb as *the* remedy for the poison-ivy dermatitis and itch is Sweet Fern. The stems and leaves are collected in the Fall and dried. When needed, a large handful of the ground herb is vigorously boiled in a quart of hot water for 2 minutes. When cool, the decoction is strained and applied to the affected area every hour as needed.

Soap Suppository: Cut a piece of Castille or Ivory-type soap to measure about ¼ by 1¼ inch. Smooth the corners until the piece is a cone and properly shape one end for insertion. When needed, the bullet-shaped suppository is oiled with a little Olive Oil or other vegetable oil and inserted. However, one must be sure to enemate the rectum with water to completely eliminate all traces of the soap.

❧   ❧   ❧

SODIUM BICARBONATE

This chemical, long fallen into deserved disuse, will like so many other harmful drugs, also be soon exiled to the therapeutic limbo "unwept and unhonored and unsung." True, at one time it had been used in medicine to counteract the acidity of the stomach or urine and in half to one teaspoonful doses had been taken to help ease discomfort of acid indigestion or heartburn which possible therapeutic benefits are greatly to be discounted and its consideration for internal purposes entirely rejected.

The medical laity has finally accepted the oft-proven fact that the continuous use of sodium bicarbonate—or any excess of it taken as an internal remedy—greatly contributed to the condition known as alkalosis. Such a condition is one "in which the blood is unduly alkaline, the equilibrium between its acids and bases being displaced in favor of the latter; it is marked by slow pulse, dizziness and a jerky state of the muscles," as quoted from Stedman's *Medical Dictionary*.

However, it may be used as a gargle, mouth and nose wash: A teaspoonful dissolved in a half glass of water, it is claimed, "leaves your mouth feeling clean and fresh."

The manufacturer of one brand of sodium bicarbonate says that since it meets all the requirements of the United States Pharmacopoeia and is acceptable to the American Dental Association, Council on Dental Therapeutics, for use as a dentifrice for both natural and artificial teeth, it may be used to clean teeth and help "prevent the growth of acid-forming bacteria that may cause tooth decay. . . ." A weak solution of the soda becomes a dentifrice by dissolving ¼-⅓ teaspoonful in ½ glass of warm water.*

Externally, a solution (4 tablespoonsful dissolved in 6 or 7 ounces of water) serves as a jiffy dressing for minor burns which is purported to "alleviate the pain and encourage recovery."

Today, as in 1840, when the following passage was written, it may provide a fair antidote for bee stings: "Bind on the place, a thick paste of saleratus moistened; it will soon extend the Venom." Temporary relief for a mild attack of hives may be obtained by hourly applications of a warm solution of the chemical using 2 teaspoonsful to a glass of hot water. Follow each application with a liberal dusting of talcum or baby powder.

An excellent, practical use for sodium bicarbonate is its cleansing properties, "cleanses refrigerators as recommended by leading refrigerator manufacturers." This cleansing effect is suitable also for glass coffee makers and thermos jugs.

Remember: In cooking of vegetables, *add no sodium bicarbonate to any food* to better preserve the B and C vitamins; if necessary, heat or better steam them in as little water as possible. The addition of an alkaline substance like soda will further the destruction of large amounts of these and other nutrients. The chemical is generally added to over-cooked, fading foods merely to preserve the color, hardly to preserve any of the much-needed chlorophyll-plus nutrients.

For insect or spider bites: Apply a wet compress of cold vinegar in which the chemical has been dissolved. Use a heaping teaspoonful to a cup.

❧   ❧   ❧

SOYA

Dr. G. Findley Stines tells us that the Soyas are heavily loaded with proteins and minerals, and pound for pound, he states, the beans have twice as much protein as beefsteak has. On

---

* Note: A proprietary tooth-paste Dentosol, contains sodium bicarbonate and glycerine and is flavored with Peppermint.

the same basis, your milk and eggs cost about 10 times as much as soya flour. When soya is used as a "food-stretcher," that is, added to the soups and foods that you like, it increases their nutritional value and cuts their cost. Dr. Stines says:

Another of Soya's valuable properties is its high alkalinity, being about 20 times more alkaline than milk. And it is loaded with minerals too—calcium, phosphorus, sodium, potassium, magnesium, sulphur, iron, zinc and copper. Its protein portion is rich in the essential amino acids; and the bean has recently been used in large quantities as the basic source of rare sterols, used in making hormones and like substances, such as the new anti-arthritic wonder drugs.

Soya is rich in oil but contrary to the natural assumption it is not fattening. It is rich in lecithin, which is one of our most important fat transporters within the body. Unlike wheat flour, soya contains an infinitesimal amount of starch. In making bread, it should constitute not more than one part to eight parts of wholewheat flour. This permits the soya to add its rich store of calcium, protein and vitamins to the wheat and still make a well-textured finished bread of good color and balance.

One of Soya's most important values as a food for infants is its high content of linoleic acid and linolenic acids, the unsaturated fatty acids so essential in promoting healthy skin tissue. In fact it has been shown that soybean oil in emulsified form has actually corrected many severe cases of infantile eczema, when due to dietary deficiency of these unsaturated acids. For such purposes only the pure pressed oil is used; because, unlike that prepared for salad oils, it contains all of the valuable acids, vitamins and lecithin.

You can easily grow your own soya bean sprouts in a four-by-five apartment . . . a milk-bottle full in five days. Skinned, steamed for 10 minutes and then chilled, they are excellent in salads and aspics. Cooked in soups or added to meat or spaghetti casseroles, they give a fresh nutty flavor that is delicious.

Soy Beans being a legume require slow cooking to render them more digestible. It is best to soak them for several hours, or even overnight, before heat is applied. To bring out the true, rich flavor, cook them in the least amount of water and in a stainless double boiler.

The Soy Beans contains about 35% proteins, 20% fat and

very little starch; of minerals, there are potassium, phosphorus, magnesium and small amounts of calcium and iron.

Sprouted Grains for the Relief of Common Ailments

The daily use of Sprouted Seeds has been found beneficial in relieving such painful and all too prevalent conditions as Arthritis, Neuritis, Rheumatism, Stiff Joints, Constipation and many other chronic complaints. It is well to bear in mind that such so-called "diseases" are only the result of *MALNUTRITION* and *TOXIC POISON*. Giving them a name does not alter this truth. The name of a complaint or disease is not important. Our desire is to be rid of it. By supplying the body with the essentials needed to feed the cells, Nature will do her own restoration work.

Sprouted Seeds have the elements needed to stimulate cell growth, also give a higher Vitamin and Mineral value to the body. The use of Sprouted Seeds is being advocated more and more as a means of better nutrition, as well as a source of food that has not been poisoned with spray. A special effort should be made to use them more abundantly each day.

All of the minerals and vitamins are at their highest peak of activity, during the sprouting period. Because of this, there would be a much greater value of both the mineral and vitamin content in the seeds at this time.   *Dr. Hazel R. Parcells.*

🌷   🌷   🌷

STRAWBERRY

"A pot of Strawberries gathered in the Wood
to mingle with your cream."   *Ben Johnson.*

Dr. William Meyrick quotes from a contemporary herbal physician, Dr. (Digitalis) Withering: "The fruits are grateful, cooling and something acid, and when taken in large quantities, they seldom disagree, they promote perspiration and dissolve tartareous incrustation of the teeth. People afflicted with the gout or stone have frequently been relieved by using (eating) them regularly." And although Herbalist Culpepper believed that the fruits of this plant were "singularly good for the healing of many ills," it was Linnaeus, the famous Swedish botanist, who first proved, after many experiments, that these berries were an excellent remedy—or a near cure—for gout and rheumatic disorders.

Many were (and still are) the medicinal properties attributed to the ripened fruits: Herbalist Gerard (1597) claimed that eaten whole they "quench thirst and take away, if they be often used, the redness and heate of the body." He was not alone in claiming that a decoction of the leaves and fruits "strengthneth the gummes and fastneth the teeth." The virtues of the fruits are further extolled, being recommended for such people who eat too much and for bleared men who have obscured vision due to a watery discharge.

And Herbalist Bancke further claimed "it (the fruit) is good to destroy the web in a man's eyes."

The Indians called it the "heart" berry from its shape and color. They made preserves of them and dried them for winter use. They also used the roots to make a tea for stomach complaints, especially for babies and young children.

Yes, indeed, the herbalist considers fresh Strawberries a valuable dentifrice, an almost perfect means of preventing tartar (the tartareous incrustation) to settle on the teeth. Cut in half, the fruit is rubbed over the tartar-covered teeth, and for best results, the juice must remain on the teeth for as long as possible and then be rinsed with a little warm water.

To remove the discoloration caused by sunburn, dab the area with a little of the juice distilled with warm water.

The fruits are easily digested and should be consumed in cupful amounts to help relieve a minor urinary disorder, kidney stone, etc. Liberal amounts should also be eaten in cases of poor complexion, skin disorders, acne, etc., and wherever a toxin-eliminant is indicated. The blood cleansing property of Strawberries is due to their high proportion of Vitamin C, malic and citric Acids, and minerals of sulfur, silicon, calcium, potassium and iron.

If you are fortunate enough to find any plants growing wild or being cultivated by a friendly farmer, by all means do collect and dry them, later to use the ground, dried leaves as a healthful substitute for pekoe tea. M-m-m, wholesome and refreshing! It is easily prepared by steeping a teaspoonful in a cup of hot water for 10 minutes, stirring and straining. The properties of the tisane are those of the fruits, although it possesses no Vitamin C.

Strawberries, in the view of a Czechoslovakian medical

writer, have a beneficial effect on disorders of the intestinal
tract, liver, heart and kidney. As *Apothecary* has reported,
A. T. Tasev recommends strawberries in some internal diseases, in the journal *Ceskoslovenska Gastroenterolocie a
Vyziva*, published in Prague. He commends strawberries in
particular favorable influence to their content of sugar, organic acids, vitamins, potassium, pectin and a small amount
of fine fiber.

❧   ❧   ❧

SUGAR

It is the opinion of most nutritionists and hygienists that white
sugar is not only a deceptive and destructive food; it acts as
Dr. Herbert Shelton says, as a

dangerously vicious poison, having been deprived of its basic,
nutritional values; and in addition because of its composition,
leaches out of the system the nutritive elements present there.
Especially does refined sugar rob the vital calcium of the teeth,
bones, and blood often resulting in such organic disorders as
nervousness, decayed teeth, diabetes, etc. It is important to remember that since much of the sugar is quickly absorbed from the
intestinal tract, eating large quantities of it may overwhelm the
ability of the liver to withdraw the sugar from the blood and may
lead to hyperglycemia and the appearance of glucose in the urine,
a condition known as alimentary glycosuria.

It is therefore recommended that one who seeks better
health should consume a minimum of such foodless, commercialized food items as candy, canned foods, soft drinks, ice
cream, cakes, custard, and especially soft drinks. On the
other hand, these sources of natural sugar should be used:
Honey—the ambrosia of the gods, unsulfured molasses, and
Raw Brown Sugar. However, the pharmacist employs sugar
in the manufacturing of a variety of preparations: Syrups,
tablets, troches, capsules, powders, etc. Sugar is also employed to render oils miscible with water, to cover the taste
of medicines and to give pharmaceutical preparations consistency.

Brown sugar, if raw and unprocessed, contains the vital

nutritive values which the healthless white variety lacks. It, therefore, becomes a worthy ally for the kitcheneer not only as food but as an ingredient in a variety of medicinal remedies. Its use is suggested in the making of cough lozenges or drops and candied roots and leaves.

Cough Syrup: Ingredients—Anise seed (or Mint), Boneset, Coltsfoot, Hoarhound, Hollyhock Root (or Mallow), Mullein and Thyme. (See also under Rosemary). Use equal parts of any combination and mix. Slowly simmer an ounce of the mixture in a pint of boiling water for 20 minutes, the utensil being covered. Stir and strain. To each cupful of liquid, add 1⅓ cup of sugar. Stir well until completely dissolved. Strain into a clean bottle and cover. The dose is a dessertspoonful sipped slowly, as often as is needed to allay irritation due to a cough or cold.

Herbal Lozenge: Anise-seeds, Coltsfoot, Currants, Hoarhound, Hollyhock or Marshmallow Roots, Mullein Leaves, Sassafras Bark and Thyme. Use 2 cups of the herb or a mixture of herbs, freshly dried and ground, 1 quart of boiling water and 4-5 cups of brown sugar.

Preparation: To prepare your own cough drops or lozenges, you may follow the general procedure for making molasses candy, or for making Hoarhound drops. Boil the herb briskly in the water about 10 minutes and simmer another 30 minutes. Stir well and strain through cheese cloth. Add about 1½ cups of the sugar to each cupful of the strained decoction and boil again. Stir until the solution begins to thicken. The mixture is then poured onto a buttered pan and cut in squares, while it is cooling. The squares when dry are powdered with a minimum of confectionary sugar.

Mr. James P. Ronald, member of the Museum Herb Club and expert on the manufacture of medicinal lozenges, uses these ingredients for his compound Hoarhound drops: Hoarhound, Hollyhock roots, Orange Peel, Mullein, Licorice, Ginger, Thyme and Mint.

When making a lozenge of Anise or some other *aromatic* herb, always first prepare the tea of herbs of your choice, Boneset, Mallow, Mullein, and then add the aromatic when ready to simmer another 30 minutes. Keep the utensil covered during the cooking process.

Note: In the preparation of Hoarhound candy or Lozenges,

Anise, Angelica Root, Cinnamon, Ginger, and Mint may be included. Use only porcelain or stainless steel utensils.

"Sugar-Eaters, BEWARE: We'd all be better off if sugar had never been discovered as a human food."

    Dr. Clive M. McCoy, Top Nutritionist at Cornell University.

"It should be prohibited by law as the drug heroin is prohibited."   *Dr. Daniel T. Quigley,*

    Lee Nutrition Foundation, Milwaukee, Wisc.

"Natural sugars mean natural energy and natural health. The day will come when this nation will tear itself from the octopus of commercialized sugars. When that day comes, there will be a new race born, free from tooth trouble, free from diabetes, and with an inexhaustible energy."   *Paul C. Bragg.*

Sugar eats the calcium in the teeth and other structures, which results in decayed teeth, nervousness and hysteria. Women generally have a deficiency of calcium because of the excess of sugar and candy, ice-cream and such sweet items that they constantly eat. . . . When the sugar is in the stomach, it takes up the calcium from other foods and the blood is thus robbed of the needed calcium. Eating candies, sweets and starches, and especially among children, is simply robbing the system of the valuable calcium.

    Sweet to the taste is bitter to the stomach;
    Bitter to the taste is sweet to the stomach.

SPRY

See under Ointment Bases.

SUMMER SAVORY

The culinary properties of Summer Savory cannot be lightly discussed, without expressing the dual role which is significant of all culinary herbs: The culinary represents the preventative aspect and the medicinal, the corrective. To emphasize this point, we will take for granted that Savory leaves and tops are used in soups and stews, meat dishes and salads, etc., but the reason for the inclusion of this herb in any recipe is purely a matter of *preventing future serious organic ailments*. To certain coarse, fatty or oily foods as meat or fish (and therefore highly cholesterolized), Savory will offer the beneficial essence of its aromatic volatile oil which in many cases tends to correct and prevent a possible dangerous catarrhal inflamed condition in the intestines (as colitis). And as a result, it will be found that its medicinal actions, as a carminative and stimulating aromatic, will be of great catarrh-preventing benefit to the digestive irregularities.

But on the other hand, if not more important, the vigorously alkalizing principle of this herb is of excellent service in preventing the artery-hardening cholesterol from causing too much damage to the blood stream. (Then why eat such second-hand foods at all?)

The average user of herbs or at least the kitcheneer should carefully evaluate the medicinal values of friend Savory. True, the present day herb-user will no doubt disagree with, yes, even ridicule, the non-"scientific" writings of Nicholas Culpepper who, like so many of his contemporaries, was wont to overpraise, though unintentionally, the more favorable qualities of any and all herbs, of culinary or medicinal nature. According to Mr. Culpepper "the juice (or a diluted infusion of Savory leaves) dropped into the eyes removes dimness of sight if it proceeds from thin humours distilled from the brain. The juice heated with oil of Roses and dropped in the ears removes noise and singing and deafness (i.e., earache), outwardly applied with wheat flour it gives ease to them." And again he reminds us that Savory "expels tough phlegm from the chest and lungs, quickens the dull spirits in the lethargy; if the juice be snuffed up the nose, dropped in the eye, it clears them of cold humours proceeding from the brain; outwardly applied with wheat flour poultice, it eases sciatica and palsied members."

To justify Mr. Culpepper's remarks, one need but to review the following medicinal properties of the herb: A warm infusion of the leaves will often correct a severe case of flatulence or wind colic, for which it is considered by some writers a specific remedy. When drunk warm, this infusion is most beneficial in feverish colds. Savory adds its aromatic and taste-disguising qualities to a typical combination of such bitterish herbs as Yarrow and Boneset, with the result that this worthy trio becomes more acceptable as an excellent "cold breaker" to the neophyte user of herb mixtures.

The Savory infusion, drunk cold either alone or with the Yarrow and Boneset, acts as a gentle but thorough tonic after a siege of cold or cough, or both. The volatile oil of Summer Savory has been used to relieve the pain of toothache and applied to the tooth cavities in manner similar to Clove Oil. However, whenever there is indicated an inflammation of the gums or the tooth area, the following mixture may be employed as a poultice to reduce the fever and symptoms: Finely ground Hop—1 part, Ground Sassafras—2 parts, finely ground Savory—1 part. Of this mixture, ½-⅔ teaspoonful contained in muslin cloth, is steeped in hot water, and applied directly to the affected area. Apply every half hour for the best results.

Note: The three herbs in a Poloris Dental Poultice are Capsicum (Red Pepper), Hops and Sassafras.

Anti-Colic Remedy: Savory, Catnip and Mint of each equal parts. Stir, strain, and drink one such cupful every 2 to 3 hours, as needed.

Diaphoretic Remedy: In colds and fevers: Mix equal parts of the above mixture, plus one of Boneset and Sage, or ½ teaspoonful of all in a cup of hot water. Prepare and drink a cupful as before.

❦   ❦   ❦

Modern Food

The public subsist upon food which, originally grown on soil poisoned with chemical fertilizers has been preserved, dehydrated, devitalized, heated, frozen, tinned, painted with creosote, strained with cochineal, or otherwise treated until its nutritive value is similar to that of the salt horse of sailing ship days.

The comparatively new idea of dehydrating food has certainly got the ancient Egyptians beaten at their own game of mummification.

The idea is simple: Refine, condense, and dehydrate the stuff. Seal it up in cardboard, transport it a few thousand miles over the sea. Keep it in a stuffy shop for a few months, then open it up, add water, and finally cook it again to make quite sure any life-giving properties that might have survived are killed.

N. Burchett.

🌷 🌷 🌷

TAMARIND

This handsome tree, although indigenous to tropical Africa, is also found throughout the eastern Mediterranean countries, India and Indonesia and has been naturalized in upper South America, the West Indies, Mexico and lower California. The fruits were well known to the early Arabian physicians who are credited with being the first to employ them both as food and as medicine.

How true it is, when one considers the basic values of vegetable medicines, that "it would be better if the modern physicians were more familiar with the grateful home-made drink that Tamarinds afford the parched sufferer with fever." Tamarinds have since early times been used in their native lands in the preparation of a refrigerant, a cooling, medicinal drink, which is much relished by those afflicted with high fevers. This febrifugal action is due to such fruit acids as citric, tartaric and malic which together with the potassium bitartrate content also causes a mildly laxative action. However, in the West Indies where it is eaten as an everyday food, it is much used as a diuretic and as a remedy for bilious disorders. And so we find in the writings of an early Colonial physician: "The pulp of Tamarinds is an agreeable laxative acid substance of great use in both putrid and inflammatory disorders for abating heat and thirst, correcting putrefaction and keeping the belly soluble; it operates also by urine, and is serviceable in the jaundice."

Pulp of Tamarind: Wash a few of the fruits in cold water and digest them in a small quantity of warm water. Then pass them through a sieve.

Electuary of Tamarind: Of the pulp take 1½ ounces, of Raspberries or Strawberries and of Honey 1 ounce each, and mix well. Take two teaspoonsful morning and night as a laxative.

Infusion of Tamarind: In a quart of boiling water, infuse for one hour, an ounce of the pulp and strain when tepid, drink slowly half a cup diluted with a little water every 2 or 3 hours. This cooling drink is much used in the warmer climates as a fever breaker.

🌷   🌷   🌷

TEA

Tea drinkers should not discard their once used Tea bags but should save them for a future need, so that in an emergency the tannic acid content of the leaves may perform a worthy service. As a lotion for a recent scalding or minor burns, the leaves, either loose or in bags, should be strongly decocted in boiling water for 10 or 15 minutes, three bags to a pint of water. The decoction when allowed to cool completely, is applied to the affected area as a compress. The healing effect is most satisfactory.

A Tea infusion when weakly diluted, has been used as a home remedy for sore and irritated eyes. It has been reported to me that the dilution of a teaspoonful of the tea solution to ⅔ cup of water has been of especial benefit as an eyedrop to long-suffering hay-feverites. The latter may also steep Rose petals (which see) in the recently infused solution of Tea until cool.

For summer complaints (diarrhea, etc.) a tablespoonful of the warm Tea solution and one of boiled, warm milk, to which is added a sprinkle of Cinnamon is quite efficacious when one such dose is drunk every ½ to 1 hour until 4 doses are taken. (However, do not give Tea to children: see under Milk.)

Attention should again be given to the Poison Antidote which calls for Tea, Toast and Magnesia. And here again, the tannic acid of the Tea is of decided benefit, to counteract any alkaline poison.

Although Dr. Meyrick had noted that several of his medical contemporaries were prescribing green Tea as a diuretic, he objected most severely to its being eaten alone or with other foods and stated in part: "I have lately observed several young ladies eat large quantities of neat green Tea, with the greatest apparent relish imaginable; whatever can induce them to follow so absurd a practice I know not, but I can assure them it is *exceedingly pernicious when so taken."*

🌱 🌱 🌱

"There is nothing with which man has to do that is of more importance than a knowledge of food, its composition, preparation, and effect upon the body; its good as well as bad effects, its conversion into brain and brawn. For it has all to do with health, and without health nothing can be accomplished."

Dr. John H. Tilden.

🌱 🌱 🌱

THYME

To mention the more practical kitchen uses of this herb, reminds me of John Parkinson's famous words regarding Thyme and its various possibilities:

To set down all the particular uses whereunto Thyme is applied were to weary both writer and Reader. I will but note only but a few; for beside the physical uses to many purposes for the head, stomach, spleen, etc., there is no herbe almost of more use, in the houses of high and low, rich and poore, both for inward and outward occasions; outwardly for bathing among hot herbs, and among other sweet herbs for strewings; inwardly in most sorts of broth (soup); with Rosemary, to make sauce for diverse sorts of both fish and flesh, as to stuffe the belly of a Goose to bee roasted and after put into the sauce, on meat when it is roasted or fried fish. It is held by divers others to bee a speedy remedy against the sting of a Bee, being bruised and layd thereone.

The oil of Thyme according to *The Dispensatory* is *"powerfully germicidal."* The derivation of Thyme will help to emphasize the usage of the herb: It is taken from the Latin *fumus* meaning to smoke, fume or steam, and from the Greek word *thymiand* (sacrifice) suggesting an herb used as incense to perfume or disinfect the temples.

"But if a pinching winter thou forsee
And would'st preserve thy famished family
With fragrant Thyme the city fumigate."

Thus we may discover that the reason for including Thyme with Rosemary and other herbs in disinfecting a sickroom (via the Incensier method) is due to the volatile oil containing Thymol and Carvacrol, the latter being the active principle also of the oil of Summer Savory. Actually it is the substance Thymol occurring in a natural state in the herb (i.e. in the volatile oil) that renders fresh Thyme as efficacious as it is. Thymol, Professor Youngken says, has been employed as an anthelmintic in the case of hook worms, as an antiseptic and deodorant in mouth washes and gargles, and occasionally as an intestinal antiseptic.

Nearly four hundred years have passed since the publication of Mr. William Turner's *Herbal,* where the use of Thyme as a remedial agent was emphasized, and its efficacy later verified by herbalists and the ever-doubting medical laity alike. Mr. Turner had noted well Thyme's ever important healing property in bronchitis, whooping cough, etc., declaring that it "hath the power to drive forth flegme." This therapeutic feature is indeed corroborated by the conservative *Dispensatory.*

The label on a bottle of Pertussin will declare that it is composed of a "Saccharated extract of Thyme"—Taeschner Method. The alcoholic extract (Thyme leaves steeped in grain alcohol) is mixed with sugar and water to form this syrup. The syrup is of benefit in whooping cough and a reasonable facsimile can be made right in your own kitchen merely by steeping or simmering wild Thyme herb in warm water, the standard remedy for centuries. Regarding the various purposes for which Thyme is intended, much has been written by many authorities of the past and present day.

No less than one of America's foremost pharmacognacists, Professor Heber W. Youngken, has for over two decades been teaching the students at the Massachusetts College of Pharmacy that the medicinal properties of garden Thyme *(T. vulgaris)* are antispasmodic, carminative and stimulant; of wild Thyme *(T. serepyllum),* antispasmodic in the treatment of whooping cough, dry nervous asthma, severe spasms where there is little sputum, and other respiratory inflammation.

Please note that this latter application as a respiratory inflammation, cold-cough remedy has been often mentioned in herbal literature past and present. Furthermore, Dioscorides in the first century, recommended Thyme (tea) mixed with honey, as a remedy for throat (bronchial) disease and asthma, and that mixture, averred John Gerard was (ed.—and still is) "good against the cough and shortness of breath." And for that condition Grandfather Isaiah mixed honey with a prepared infusion of Thyme and Linseeds (and Garlic for the asthmatic) which helped to provide lasting relief. An elderly English gentleman, an herbalist and friend, compared Thyme to Tincture Benzoin Compound (which is much used as a vaporizing inhalant): "When any of the children had a cough, Thyme was put to smoulder on a low heat, the pleasant fumes giving easier breathing."

Cough Syrup, Child's: Mix intimately one teaspoonful each (or equal parts of) Anise, Hoarhound, Irish Moss, Mallow (or Hollyhock) leaves, Licorice and wild Thyme. Simmer 2 teaspoonsful of the mixture in a pint of hot water for 10 minutes. Allow to cool for half an hour and strain. Add ½ cup of brown sugar or honey to each cupful of liquid. Dose: For children, one or two teaspoonsful every hour or two. For infants ½ to 1 teaspoonful every 2 to 3 hours.

Cough Syrup, Adults: Mix together equal parts of wild Thyme, Boneset, Hoarhound, Irish Moss, Chestnut leaves. Prepare as above. Dose: One or two teaspoonsful every ½ to 1 hour as required. Sip slowly.

Antacid: Equal parts of Fennel, Anise, Linden, Catnip, Mint, and Thyme. A teaspoonful of this mixture is steeped 5 to 7 minutes in a cupful of hot water and strained. The dose is a cupful sipped slowly as often as required, but abstaining from food for one hour previous to taking the tea.

Cough Lozenges: Use the procedure outlined under Sugar, starting with a base of equal parts of Anise, Thyme and Boneset (or others if you prefer). Simmer, do not boil the mixture.

Blood Cleanser Formula: Mix equal portions of Thyme, Watercress, Blueberry and Sassafras Bark. Directions: Steep a teaspoonful of the mixture in a cup of hot water and let stand covered until cool. Stir, strain, drink one cupful 4 times a day, abstaining from foods as much as possible.

TOMATO

The Tomato offers its optimum of nutrients *only* if it is eaten uncooked, in its nature-all, original form. The canned juice is truly a poor second. And furthermore, there is no comparison between the commercially cultivated fruit and that which you will raise via the *organic-gardening* method, without chemical and poisonous fertilizers and spray insecticides but with a great deal of loving kindness, fertilizing the soil with vegetable discards and weed-like material, and cherishing each growing plant so raised with a greater source of organicultural pride.

Remember: The fresh Tomato or/and its juice if eaten alone or with other fresh vegetables has an alkaline reaction; but when ingested with bread, crackers or other starches or sugared foods and eaten together at the same meal, will often cause an acid reaction and subsequent stomach distress.

Ayerst, McKenna and Harrison Ltd., a drug manufacturing concern of New York City, several years ago, released Tomectin, a product containing fresh dried Tomato pulp in a pectin base. According to the company's literature, Tomectin was offered for the "effective management of diarrheal conditions —(and has) been found to bring about a favorable response when other antidiarrheal medication had failed. . . . The Tomato substance in Tomectin is obtained from fresh, ripe, whole Tomatoes and not from Tomato pomace which describes a by-product of the Tomato canning industry."

Dried Tomato Pulp Works Quickly for Relief of Diarrhea: The successful use of tomato pomace in more than 100 cases of diarrhea is described by Dr. Lester M. Morrison of the Philadelphia General Hospital. In the *American Journal of Digestive Diseases,* 13: 196, 1946, he says that diarrhea from simple or non-organic cause was usually stopped within 4 hours by the tomato treatment.

The substance used in this study, prepared by tomato pulp dehydration, relieved diarrhea from food poisoning, mucous and spastic colitis, nutritional deficiencies, food allergy (other than that to tomatoes), and other causes. No toxic symptoms were observed from its use. One tablespoon of tomato pomace was added to each glass of milk, given at two-hour intervals. Within 12 hours of the first dose, the diarrhea stopped. In this way, the patient was enabled to undergo Sippy milk diet, and within one week, ulcer symptoms disappeared. In the course of this study, it was noted that such gastric disturbances as heartburn, nausea, vomiting and belching, were often relieved promptly by the tomato pomace.

TURNIP

Did you know that the early fresh root cut into thin strips, may be eaten like an Apple? That a century ago, the roots were considered an excellent tooth cleanser if eaten uncooked and thoroughly chewed? That the leaves of this vegetable should be collected, not discarded, and prepared as a cooked vegetable, steamed for 25-30 minutes? That from this food, a group of Boston scientists has isolated and identified a substance that suppresses thyroid activity?

This fine, flavorful root possesses a most delectable odor that is due to the large percentage of sulfur, and therefore must not be prepared with high heat or in much boiling water; do slow-steam this food in the smallest amount of water for about 15 minutes, or less. The other important minerals are calcium, chlorine, magnesium, phosphorus, postassium, and sodium. One health authority believes that since Turnip leaves contain a very high percentage of calcium and potassium, they are an excellent food for growing children. (And surely for aging adults.)

A friend has suggested, that the fresh juice of Carrots and Dandelions be taken with an equal amount of Turnip juice to facilitate the hardening of soft bones and teeth. This combination, he claims, is to be taken 3 times a day in a cupful dose, and furnishes a superior source of calcium and magnesium which are so very necessary to strengthen and give firmness to the structure of all bone (tooth) formation. Another health enthusiast advocates this combination of salad foods as a preventative of and as a dietary treatment for brittle nails and falling hair: Carrots, Cabbage, Celery, Rutabaga and Turnip, a small salad for lunch and a much larger one for dinner. And a writer in a present-day herb journal believed that to clear up skin rashes and pimples common in springtime, "grated Turnip and grated Onion, plus finely chopped Carrot and a level teaspoonful of Aniseed (powder), should be mixed together and taken 3 times a day."

In early Colonial days, a syrup or decoction was much employed in the treatment of throat and bronchial disorders. It was claimed that "the decoction of Turnip is good against the cough and hoarseness of the voice, being drunk in the evening with a little sugar or honey." A more recent medical authority had written that a syrup prepared by boiling two large roots, cut in small pieces, in 2 pints of boiling water and adding an equal amount of honey to any portion of the cooled, strained liquid, is useful in coughs, hoarseness and other asthmatic disorders.

❧   ❧   ❧

VASELINE

See under Ointment Bases. Try to obtain the cheaper Petroleum Jelly.

❧   ❧   ❧

VINEGAR

The virtues of Vinegar as a seasoning agent are well known although it should be emphasized that to prepare an herb vinegar for table use, only the Malt or Cider varieties should be used. In *Better Health with Culinary Herbs,* I have outlined a few of the simple remedies that have been tried out at home with relative success.

Here for instance is an Aromatic Vinegar that should be used as an application to bites or stinging of insects, bees and to scratches, hives, bruises, etc.

Aromatic Vinegar: 1. Cinnamon, Cloves, Ginger, Lemon Peel, Orange Peel, Sassafras and Vinegar—8 ounces.

Allow one level teaspoonful of each spice to steep in the vinegar for 10 days. Stir occasionally; then stir, strain and add enough vinegar to measure 8 ounces. (If this preparation is for external use only, add 8 ounces of alcohol in which ½ ounce of Camphor has been dissolved.)

2. *Gargle:* Vinegar—1 part (or ounce), Honey—4 parts, Barley Water—4 parts. Mix and gargle every hour. The Barley water must be freshly prepared.

3. *Sunburn Remedy:* Vinegar, Olive Oil. Mix equal parts. Shake well and use before and after. ·

4. *Liniment:* Ground Cloves, Ground Ginger, Ground Red Pepper—1 tsp. of each, Turpentine—4 ounces, Vinegar—1 ounce, and Witch Hazel—3 ounces. Mix the liquids. Allow the spices to stand in the liquid for 3 or 4 days, which must be kept in a warm place. Stir and strain.

5. *Hair Application:* "Use full strength (Cider Vinegar) on the hair rubbing in a little at a time; never have used any commercial coloring on my hair." *Mrs. M.A.F.*

6. *Vinegar Cataplasm:* Flour or Corn Starch—3 parts, Vinegar—1 part. Mix well and apply to affected area. Serves well as an astringent and antiseptic application. Good for hives.

7. *Liniment of Vinegar and Turpentine:* This remedy has long been known to the pharmaceutical industry by a variety of names: St. John Long's—Stoke's—and White Liniment. It appears as an official preparation in the *National Formulary* and other medical compendia. Formula: Turpentine—7 ounces, Vinegar—2⅔ ounces, Oil of Lemon—2 teaspoonsful, Egg and Water, of each to make 16 ounces. (For Oil of Lemon may be substituted some other aromatic oil, Wintergreen, Sassafras.)

Directions: Mix the contents of one egg and the yolk of another with the turpentine and the oil until thoroughly mixed. Then add the Vinegar and half the water. Shake vigorously and add enough water to measure a pint. Be sure to shake well before using this remedy.

8. *Liniment of Vinegar and Red Pepper:* A red Pepper liniment is quickly and simply prepared by adding a heaping tablespoonful of freshly cut cayenne Peppers to a pint of warm Vinegar. Place the mixture close to or upon a warm radiator, stove or other source of heat, and allow it to stay there for an hour or so. Stir and strain. Label the bottle.

Before applying this liniment, warm the affected bruised area with warm (not hot) wet packs. For best results, gently rub in a small quantity of liniment twice an hour for 2 or 3 hours and apply a hot water bottle or a warm near-dry wet pack, or cover with heavy flannel.

❦   ❦   ❦

WALNUT

Fungicides from Walnut Husks

Black walnut and butternut shucks, shunned even by squirrels, may some day have a commercial use as producers of a fungicide, according to the Connecticut Agricultural Station at New Haven. It has long been known that soil at the base of walnut trees is toxic to higher plants, causing them to blacken and die. A few years ago the toxic chemical was isolated and called "juglone" after Juglans, the generic name of the walnut tree. Now there is a possibility the chemical may be put to work as a fungicide to combat minute parasitic forms of plant life which cause havoc with many of our food and ornamental crops.

In his search for materials to take the place of war-short copper fungicides, Dr. George A. Gries unearthed a formula concocted by a practical grower over 100 years ago. It was primarily an infusion of black walnut leaves. How successful this formula proved is not known, but it was probably considered as superstition by the scientists of the day as no further studies on it are known. The fact remains, however, that the early grower "struck the nail on the head," at least so far as the walnuts are concerned. Laboratory tests with the synthesized form of juglone prove that this material is more toxic than copper oxide.   *Horticulture.*

This article helps to prove our point: Don't ridicule the old-fashioned remedies simply because they're prepared with herbs or foods. Tomorrow they may be new-fashioned.

❧   ❧   ❧

WATERCRESS

Though the Spartans of old knew naught of the Vitamins of B Complex et al, they were quick to evaluate the efficacy of this herb's priceless ingredients, and would eat much of Watercress with their bread. They became noted for their wit and decision of character.

Watercress is an outstanding example of nature's best sources of food. It is an excellent source of Vitamin C plus A, B, E, and G. Its high vitamin C content makes it an admirable food for the elderly since the Vitamin C, especially of Watercress, will help to maintain the suppleness of the small blood vessels and thus help to ward off hardening of the arteries.

Dr. Karl Mason of Vanderbilt University has shown that the dried leaves of Watercress contained three times as much Vitamin C as the leaves of Lettuce. Furthermore, Watercress, may well boast of its content of health fortifying minerals as calcium, potassium and sodium, plus those that are constantly required to strengthen the blood stream, namely, copper, iron, manganese and sulphur.

Whenever possible, include this zesty protective food in your fresh salad and always *serve it uncooked*. And when it is included in a salad, add no other seasoning, culinary herb or vinegar. Do not cut the leaves nor incorporate it into a cole slaw.

Watercress has long enjoyed the well deserved reputation of being a blood cleanser, which therapeutic is principally due to the considerable quantity of organic sulfur and phosphorus, chlorine, et al, constituting 45% of the acid forming element. The balance includes these alkaline-forming minerals: Calcium, 18%; iron ¼%, magnesium 5%; potassium 20% and sodium 8% and other trace minerals. A formula for a "blood cleanser" remedy has already been given under Thyme.

Since Watercress is well recognized for its anti-scorbutic properties, it is indicated as a preventative or "curative" of scurvy which generally results from a diet of salt meats and a lack of fresh vegetables and fruits. The high percentage of Vitamin C contained in this food and uncooked, unpreserved fruits and vegetables is a positive factor in the healing of that still too common disease. Dr. Withering believed that the fresh leaves are very wholesome, particularly for such as are troubled with scorbutic complaints. To which, his contemporary, Dr. Meyrick adds: "It is undoubtedly an excellent antiscorbutic and stomachic and there is no better way of using it than as a salad," (i.e. uncooked). Over 200 years have passed since their days and their remarks, and these remarks are as true today as they were then.

The herbalist recommends the eating of large portions of fresh Watercress as a natural remedy in overcoming such organic ailments as dropsy and kidney disorders, jaundice, and threatening hardening of the arteries. It is also useful in the (dietary) treatment of skin and blood disorders. However, it is of the utmost importance in order to benefit the most from the ingestion of this food, to abstain from all foods for at least 2 hours prior to meal-times, and of course, to abstain from eating all artificially prepared, i.e. man-made foods, canned or packaged items, foods that are fried, boiled or salted, starches, sugars and spices, etc.

❦   ❦   ❦

WATERMELON

It seems as though it was only at yesterday's meal that Grandfather warned us not to throw away the innumerable seeds after wading through our slices of *Citrullus Vulgaris,* yes, Watermelon. Of the rinds, a culinary delicacy was soon to be composed and the necessary flavor signature to be admirably harmonized by such wild-growing seasoning spices native to New England as Wild Allspice, Sassafras and Sweet Flag.

Grandfather Isaiah, the shining example of Conservation, would save every bit of leftover that could profitably be used in the future, not that we were so frightfully poor or in such dire need of saving every morsel of food or crumb of bread, but with Grandfather saving following in line with Godliness and cleanliness. He'd save the stones or pits and stems of Cherries, the peels of Lemon and Orange, used Tea Leaves and Pumpkin seeds—yes, all of these were to be later used as medicines or for some other good use.

And, too, certain physicians here in Worcester have prescribed with most favorable results Watermelon seeds for folks who had been ailing with cardiac or heart ailments. I have learned of such beneficial results obtained by these patients who at the time of their drinking teas of ground Watermelon Seeds also suffered edema of the ankles, (that is, a painful swelling at that area).

The ritual of seed saving was no simple matter. In fact, it was quite a chore but we never questioned Grandfather's judgment. Ours was not to question why; ours was to save our respective Watermelon seeds. We were rewarded by having Grandfather relate to us some fable or bit of folklore pertaining to the herbs of our immediate neighborhood.

When saving Watermelon seeds for future use, dip them via a metal strainer in a mild solution of cold soapy water. The seeds dry best if first they are rolled in a towel to absorb most of the moisture. To dry completely they are spread out on large sheets of cardboard up in your attic or near your oil burner in the cellar.

Today, as in past years, there has been much publicity given to the symptomatic condition known as high blood pressure, which has been helped to a marked degree by drinking teas of Watermelon seeds. However, we must always remember that high blood pressure is not a disease in itself, but a symptom, or better perhaps, a warning that a more serious and dangerous organic condition exists. Thus, we find that an extract of watermelon seeds contains an active ingredient called Cucurbocitrin which has been of great value in dilating the capillaries or very small blood vessels. By directing its benefits toward the kidney organs, the pressure upon the large blood vessels is reduced.

Note: Watermelon should always be eaten *between meals,* or at least one hour after meals. *Never eat Melon with your meal.*

This food is a good source of quickly assimilable minerals of calcium, magnesium, phosphorus, and postassium; of Vitamins A, C, and B (thiamine).

On October 31, 1952, the newspapers carried an Associated Press story and wirephoto of a youngster who virtually held his life in his hands. The photo shows George Botot, Jr., age 8 of St. Clairsville, Ohio, flashing "a smile as he grasps one of the watermelons which may save his life. George is suffering from nephritis, a kidney disease, in which vitamins are supplied by melon combat. Appeals have resulted in three carloads of melons and more have been promised."

Melon for Sick Child

Diane Rush, 7, of Greenville, S. C. bites into a whopping slice of precious out-of-season watermelon at her home after the melon was prescribed as a possible aid in the child's fight against nephrosis, described as a relatively rare kidney disease. The child's physician told the parents that there was nothing to lose by trying watermelon, so arrangements were made to fly this and other melons in from Cuba where a small crop is now in season.

News Report.

Watermelon Seed Tea: Crush 2 teaspoonsful of the dried seeds via a meat grinder or mortar and pestle. Steep the

ground seeds in a cup of hot water for an hour. Stir and
strain. Drink one such cupful 4 times a day.

❦   ❦   ❦

WHEAT

Furacin, The Wonder Drug: Discovery that an inexpensive
drug seems to act like the wonder hormone ACTH was
announced to the American College of Surgeons. The drug,
an old one named Furacin may become a plentiful new medicine against arthritis, rheumatic fever and perhaps some kinds
of cancer. Tests on humans are just starting. Furacin is
derived from furfural, a by-product in milling flour and soy-
beans. The new discovery is that furacin apparently prods
the adrenal glands to produce cortisone.

New Vitamin Believed to Fight Infection

A "probable" new vitamin which may help human beings resist
infection was reported today by Dr. Howard A. Schneider of the
Rockefeller Research Foundation. Found in wheat, the discovery
is "probably a new nutritional" substance, Dr. Schneider told the
American Public Health Association. It has not yet been isolated
or identified, he said. The discovery was made during an eight-year
study with mice. Dr. Schneider said it showed *diet can influence
natural resistance to infectious diseases.* (My italics). Mice fed
with the new substance, he reported, showed such a resistance.

News Report.

(See under Oat).

If wheat you are to eat,
Be sure that the original *eat*
Is left in the Wheat.

Instead of eating wheat germ, why not eat the *whole* unprocessed food?

Be sure that your Wheat has a nature-all organically raised
background.

❦   ❦   ❦

Pennies for a Day's Supply of Vitamin A or Vitamin C:
U.S. Department of Agriculture researchers have figured out
how much—or rather how little—it costs to buy a day's supply of vitamin A or vitamin C in the form of fruits and
vegetables. *For only three cents* one can buy all the vitamin A
needed for a day from carrots, collards or sweet potatoes at
19 cents a pound. For four cents the same supply is obtained
from trimmed kale or spinach at 25 cents a pound or winter
squash at 25 cents. Or, for twelve cents, one can buy a day's
supply from broccoli at 35 cents a pound. It would cost 15
cents to obtain the same vitamin A supply from cantaloupe
at 25 cents a pound.

When it comes to vitamin C, *six cents buys a day's supply*
from cabbage or oranges at 15 cents a pound. Or the same
quantity of vitamin C is obtained for nine cents from grapefruit at 15 cents a pound; while ten cents buys the daily quota
from broccoli at 35 cents a pound or trimmed kale at 25
cents. Or if you prefer your vitamin C from strawberries, 15
cents would get you a day's supply when the fruit is 49 cents
a pound. And when potatoes are 10 cents a pound, 14 cents'
worth provides the desired vitamin C.

Therapeutic Uses

ACNE: *Charcoal*

ANEMIA: *Watercress*

ANT POWDER: *Borax, Fennel, Red Pepper*

ANTACID: *Anise, Caraway, Dill, Marjoram, Thyme*

ANTHELMINTIC: *See Worm Expellant*

ANTI-COLIC: *Anise, Caraway, Catnip, Cinnamon, Fennel, Savory*

ANTI-SCORBUTIC: *Cabbage, Watercress*

ANTISPASMODIC: *Catnip, Cumin*

ARTHRITIS: *Cherry, Wheat*

ASTHMA: *Cherry, Garlic, Honey, Onion, Rosemary*

BALDNESS: *Garlic, Rosemary*

BANDOLINE: *Quince*

BEDWETTING: *Honey*

BEE STING: *Sodium Bicarbonate, Vinegar*

BILIARY STONE: *Raspberry*

BITES, INSECT: *Vinegar*

BLOOD CLEANSER: *Cranberry, Thyme, Watercress*

BLOOD PRESSURE, HIGH: *Rice, Watermelon*

BOIL: *Fig, Onion*

BRONCHITIS: *Barley, Compound Tincture Benzoin, Currant, Rosemary, Thyme*

BRUISE: *Oregano, Salt, Vinegar*

BURNS: *Aloe, Butter, Cod Liver Oil, Egg, Honey, Irish Moss, Lanolin, Olive Oil, Tea, Potato, Sodium Bicarbonate*

CANKER: *Pomegranate, Sage*

CARMINATIVE: *Allspice, Anise, Catnip, Cinnamon, Clove, Coriander, Cumin, Dill, Fennel, Oregano*

CATAPLASM: *See Poultice*

CATARRH: *Fig, Sage*
CHILBLAIN: *Camphor*
COLDS: *Catnip, Ginger, Grapefruit, Raspberry, Sage, Savory*
COLIC: *Anise, Caraway, Catnip, Cinnamon, Dill, Fennel,
     Savory*
CONSTIPATION: *Fig, Soap*
CORN: *Castor Oil*
COUGH: *Anise, Cherry, Honey, Irish Moss, Milk, Okra,
     Quince, Rosemary, Sugar, Thyme, Turnip*
CRAMPS: *Ginger*

DANDRUFF: *Lemon*
DENTIFRICE: *Soap, Sodium Bicarbonate, Strawberry, Turnip*
DEODORIZER: *Cinnamon, Clove, Rosemary, Thyme*
DIABETIC RETINITIS: *Buckwheat*
DIAPHORETIC: *Catnip, Saffron, Sage, Savory*
DIARRHEA: *Apple, Blackberry, Cinnamon, Ginger, Milk, Nut-
     meg, Persimmon, Pomegranate, Raspberry, Tea, Tomato*
DIGESTANT: *Papaya*
DISINFECTANT: *Rosemary (See Deodorizer)*
DIURETIC: *Artichoke, Asparagus, Cucumber, Corn Silk, Cran-
     berry, Grape, Parsley, Parsnip, Strawberry, Watercress,
     Watermelon*
DROPSY: *Asparagus, Watercress*
DYSPEPSIA: *Charcoal, Cinnamon, Sage*

EAR: *Olive Oil, Peach*
ECZEMA: *Salt, Milk, Potato*
EMETIC: *Salt*
EMOLLIENT: *Okra*
ENEMA: *Soap, Corn Starch*
EYE LOTION: *Borax, Camphor, Fennel, Milk, Rose, Tea*

FEVER: *Catnip, Pomegranate, Potato, Raspberry, Saffron,
     Sage, Savory, Tamarind*
FEVER, HAY: *Tea*
FLATULENCE: *Anise, Caraway, Cinnamon, Dill, Fennel*
FLEA POWDER: *Fennel*
FRECKLE: *Cream, Lemon*
FUMIGANT: *Rosemary*

GALL BLADDER: *Radish*

GARGLE: *Cinnamon, Currant, Fig, Milk, Persimmon, Pomegranate, Rosemary, Sage, Sodium Bicarbonate, Vinegar*

GOUT: *Cherry, Strawberry*

HAIR: *Castor Oil, Olive Oil, Peach, Quince, Rosemary, Sage*

HALITOSIS: *Anise, Rosemary*

HAND LOTION: *Compound Tincture Benzoin, Cucumber, Irish Moss, Lanolin, Quince*

HAY FEVER: *Tea*

HEADACHE: *Basil, Marjoram, Rosemary*

HIVES: *Sodium Bicarbonate*

INDIGESTION: *Anise, Fennel, Papaya*

INSECT BITES: *Vinegar*

INSECT REPELLENT: *Red Pepper*

IVY, POISON: *Soap*

KIDNEY DISORDER: *Artichoke, Asparagus, Corn Silk, Parsley, Strawberry, Watercress, Watermelon*

LARYNGITIS: *Compound Tincture Benzoin*

LAXATIVE: *Date, Fig, Oat, Prunes, Tamarind*

LINIMENT: *Camphor, Egg, Red Pepper, Soap, Vinegar*

LIVER: *Anise*

MEASLES: *Catnip, Marjoram, Saffron*

MOTH PREVENTATIVE: *Rosemary*

MOUTH WASH: *Rosemary, Sage*

NAILS: *Parsnip*

NAUSEA: *Charcoal, Dill*

NEPHRITIS: *Watermelon*

NEPHROSIS: *Watermelon*

NERVINE: *Basil, Catnip, Rosemary, Sage*

NERVOUSNESS: *Celery, Marjoram, Parsnip, Rosemary (See under Nervine)*

NEURALGIA: *Oregano*

NEURITIS: *Rice*

NOSE DROPS: *Salt*

POISON ANTIDOTE: *Charcoal, Tea*

POISON IVY: *Cod Liver Oil, Soap*

POULTICE: *Ginger, Mustard, Oat, (Red and Black) Pepper, Soap*
PROSTATE GLAND: *Pumpkin*

REDUCING: *Fennel*
RHEUMATISM: *Asparagus, Basil, Lemon, Oregano, Strawberry*
RINGWORM: *Borax, Black Pepper*
RINSE FOR SHAMPOO: *Lemon*

SCALP: *Black Pepper*
SCARLET FEVER: *Saffron*
SHAMPOO: *Castor Oil, Egg, Lemon, Olive Oil*
SHAMPOO, RINSE: *Lemon*
SKIN: *Almond, Borax, Compound Tincture Benzoin, Castor Oil, Corn Starch, Honey, Lard, Lanolin, Lemon, Marigold, Potato*
SOAP SUBSTITUTE: *Almond*
SPRAINS: *Oregano, Salt, Vinegar*
SPRING TONIC: *Sage*
STOMACHIC: *Cinnamon, Coriander, Lemon, Sage, Watercress*

TAENICIDE: *Coconut, Garlic, Onion*
TAPEWORM EXPELLANT: *Pomegranate*
TARTAR REMOVER: *Apple, Raspberry, Strawberry*
THROAT, SORE: *Currant, Honey, Quince, Sage*
TOOTHACHE: *Catnip, Red Pepper, Savory*
TOOTHPOWDER: *Bread, Salt, Soap, Sodium Bicarbonate*

ULCERS: *Cabbage*
UTERINE RELAXANT: *Raspberry*

VAPORIZING CREAM: *Camphor*

WARTS: *Castor Oil*
WAVE SET: *Quince*
WINE: *Allspice, Cinnamon, Clove*
WORM EXPELLANT: *Coconut, Garlic, Onion, Pineapple, Pomegranate, Pumpkin*
WOUNDS (SKIN): *Compound Tincture Benzoin, Castor Oil, Squash, Cod Liver Oil, Sage*

Bibliography

Brown, Dr. O. Phelps, *The Complete Herbalist*, Jersey City, N.J., 1865.

Culpepper, Nicholas, *The English Physician*, London, 1826.

Esser, William L., *Dictionary of Foods*, John's Island, S.C., 1947.

Finckel, Dr. Harry, *Diet and Cook Book*, New York, The Society for Public Health Education, 1925.

Gerard, John, *Herball or Generall Historie of Plantes*, London, 1957.

Griffith, Dr. R. E., *A Universal Formulary*, Philadelphia, Blanchard & Lea, 1859.

Harris, Ben Charles, *Eat the Weeds*, Barre, 1969; *Better Health with Culinary Herbs*, Boston, 1952; "Yours for Better Health" Radio Broadcasts; and unpublished manuscripts.

Hartshorne, Henry, *The Household Cyclopedia*, Philadelphia, 1871.

Holt, Rockham, *George Washington Carver*, New York, Doubleday Doran Company, 1953.

Meyer, Joseph E., *The Herbalist*, Indiana Botanic Gardens, 1934.

Meyrick, Dr. William, *New Family Herbal*, London, 1740.

The National Formulary, American Pharmaceutical Association.

Parkinson, John, *Theatricum Botanicum*, London, 1640.

The Pharmaceutical Recipe Book, American Pharmaceutical Association, 1943.

Pope, Dr. R. D., *Raw Vegetable Juices*, privately published.

Richardson, Dr. J. G., and others, *Medicology or Home Encyclopedia of Health*, Dr. James P. Wood, ed., New York, University Medical Society, 1904.

Stedman, Thomas L., *A Practical Medical Dictionary* (12th ed.), William Wood and Company, 1934.

Turner, William, *Newe Herball,* London, 1568.

Wood, Horatio C. and Osol, Arthur, *The Dispensatory of the United States of America,* Philadelphia, J. B. Lippincott Company, 1943.

Youngken, Heber W., *Textbook of Pharmacognasy,* Philadelphia, P. Blakiston's Sons and Company, 1936.

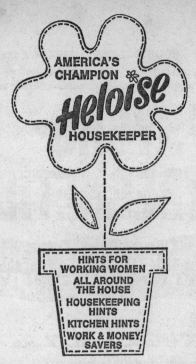

AMERICA'S CHAMPION *Heloise* HOUSEKEEPER

HINTS FOR
WORKING WOMEN
ALL AROUND
THE HOUSE
HOUSEKEEPING
HINTS
KITCHEN HINTS
WORK & MONEY
SAVERS

Hundreds of helpful hints for easier, speedier, money-saving ways to accomplish every household task.

▼ AT YOUR BOOKSTORE OR MAIL THE COUPON BELOW ▼

Mail Service Department   POCKET BOOKS   DEPT. 27
A Division of Simon & Schuster, Inc./1 W. 39th St./New York, N.Y. 10018
Please send me the following:

No. of Copies	Amount	#	Price	Title
		77371	(95¢ ea.)	Heloise's Hints for Working Women
		77372	(95¢ ea.)	Heloise All Around the House
		77373	(95¢ ea.)	Heloise's Housekeeping Hints
		77374	(95¢ ea.)	Heloise's Kitchen Hints
		77375	(95¢ ea.)	Heloise's Work and Money Savers

Plus 25¢ .... for mailing and handling
Please enclose check or money order. We are not
TOTAL AMOUNT .... responsible for orders containing cash.

(PLEASE PRINT CLEARLY)

Name...

Address...

City..State..................Zip..........................

P 33/1

Let this

FAMOUS PLASTIC SURGEON'S REMARKABLE DISCOVERY

*help you escape life's dull, monotonous routine—
make you look younger, feel healthier, be more successful!*

PSYCHO-CYBERNETICS

A New Way to GET MORE LIVING OUT OF LIFE

By

MAXWELL MALTZ, M.D., F.I.C.S.

Based on an amazing new scientific innovation,
this simple yet practical "new way of
life" can be the most important
influence in your life!

78092/$1.25

▼ AT YOUR BOOKSTORE OR MAIL THE COUPON BELOW ▼

Mail Service Department   POCKET BOOKS   DEPT. 15
*A Division of Simon & Schuster, Inc./*1 W. 39th St./New York, N.Y. 10018
Please send me the following:

No. of Copies	Amount	#	Price	Title
....	....		78092 ($1.25 each)	PSYCHO-CYBERNETICS

Plus 25¢.................... for mailing and handling

TOTAL AMOUNT .... Please enclose check or money order. We are not responsible for orders containing cash.

(PLEASE PRINT CLEARLY)

Name ....

Address ....

City.. State........................ Zip....................

P 11/1